As Far As Words Go

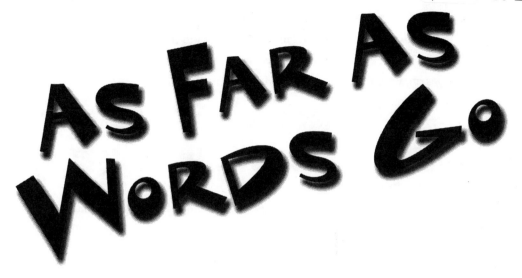

Unraveling the Complexities of Ambiguous Language and Humor

Cecile Cyrul Spector, PhD, CCC-SLP

Thinking Publications · Eau Claire, Wisconsin

11   10   09   08   07   06   05   8   7   6   5   4   3   2

Library of Congress Cataloging-in-Publication Data
      Spector, Cecile Cyrul, date.
         As far as words go / unraveling the complexities of ambiguous language and humor /
      Cecile Cyrul Spector.
                  p. cm.
         Includes bibliographical references. (p.   ).
         ISBN 1-888222-83-2 (alk. paper)
            1. Language disorders. 2. Speech therapy. 3. Play on words. 4. Ambiguity. 5. Wit and
      humor. I. Title.
      RC423 .S6348 2001
      616.85'5—dc21   2001046259

Printed in the United States of America

Cover and game mat design by Patti Argoff

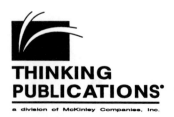

**THINKING
PUBLICATIONS®**
a division of McKinley Companies, Inc.

424 Galloway Street • Eau Claire, WI 54703
715.832.2488 • Fax 715.832.9082
Email: custserv@ThinkingPublications.com

COMMUNICATION SOLUTIONS THAT CHANGE LIVES®

For David, Rachel,
Sarah, and Stephanie
with love

About the Author

Cecile Cyrul Spector, PhD, has worked in the field of speech-language pathology for over 30 years. She received her BA and MA from Brooklyn College of the City of New York, and her PhD from New York University. She started out by providing clinical services in public schools, private practice, and at the Hofstra University clinic. Eventually she joined the faculty of Long Island University–Orangeburg Campus where for 10 years she taught a wide range of courses and was the director of the Speech-Language Department. She also taught many courses as an adjunct professor at The College of New Rochelle, Montclair State University, and New York University.

Cecile has made numerous research presentations and given workshops that have focused on various aspects of humor, ambiguity, and figurative language. Most of her journal articles have been on this same subject matter.

As a clinician, Cecile has worked with individuals from 18 months to 80-plus years. Language-learning disabled adolescents and adults who incurred brain injury as a result of strokes or accidents were the populations that sparked her interest in the subtleties of abstract language.

In addition to enjoying family-oriented activities, Cecile's other interests include cooking, reading, hiking, swimming, golf, and travel. Wherever she goes, Cecile is on the lookout for snippets of humor and ambiguity to add to her collection.

Contents

Preface

The words of language, like the notes of music, can be combined in an infinite number of ways. The potential range of meanings is awesome. The variety of meanings of many English words and the numerous ways in which they can be combined gives the language its delicious richness and complexity. It makes our conversational language a beautiful palette of subtly mixed shades, tints, and colors and allows for a more efficient use of vocabulary items. Think of how large our lexicon would be if each word were restricted to only one possible meaning!

The very factors that make language so interesting—richness and complexity—are also the characteristics that makes English so difficult for many individuals to learn. For most people, simply being exposed to the multiple meanings of words, phrases, and sentences is a sufficient condition for learning them. Unfortunately, individuals with language-learning difficulties need well-designed structure to be able to understand ambiguous language and humor. Mere exposure is not enough. *As Far as Words Go: Unraveling the Complexities of Ambiguous Language and Humor* was designed to provide such structure.

Some of the activities in *As Far as Words Go* are based on examining elements of linguistic humor, their ambiguous nature, and the figurative language that is interwoven throughout these elements. Other activities follow a more traditional academic format (e.g., defining words, matching items, and developing paragraphs). Through the activities in this resource, individuals have opportunities for increasing their vocabulary, expanding their world knowledge, enhancing their metalinguistic awareness, improving their problem-solving skills, and refining their discourse skills.

The act of "dissecting" jokes may reduce or eliminate their funniness. Not to worry! Once the ability to truly understand linguistic humor is achieved, funniness will be even greater for "undissected" humor items.

This book may be considered a companion to *Saying One Thing, Meaning Another: Activities for Clarifying Ambiguous Language* (Spector, 1997) and *Sound Effects: Activities for Developing Phonological Awareness* (Spector, 1999) in that it targets some of the same skills and uses a cognitive-strategies approach to intervention. However, *As Far As Words Go* contains new and different linguistic tasks, adds another humor category (i.e., switching words), and uses some additional intervention techniques (e.g., a game mat format).

Several important issues discussed in *Saying One Thing, Meaning Another* are relevant to the skills and techniques used in *As Far as Words Go*. The key points will be repeated, but you are encouraged to refer to *Saying One Thing, Meaning Another* to obtain additional information about these issues.

Acknowledgments

The efforts of many people helped bring this book to its present form. I am truly grateful to my editor, Angie Sterling-Orth, for "smoothing out" the "rough edges" of my original manuscript and for her patient manner. Thanks also to Nancy McKinley, Linda Schreiber, Joyce Olson, Sarah Thurs, and Heather Johnson Schmitz, who took part in the editing process; to Patti Argoff, for designing the book's cover and game mat (I asked for lots of color, and she gave me lots of color!); to Debbie Olson, who provided the book's format and whimsical graphics; and to the reviewers—Kathy Gorman-Gard, Beth Hibbard, Sue Heuselee, Marilyn Nippold, and Nancy Lund—whose comments and suggestions were used to improve the organization, scope, and quality of the introductory text and intervention activities.

It is my good fortune that my writing efforts have always been encouraged and supported by my entire family. My love and thanks to my husband, Mort, for acting as "consultant" on many facets of this book; to my sister Glady, for her editing efforts; and to my children and grandchildren, who, by their very existence, make me happy.

Part I
INTRODUCTION

Overview

As Far as Words Go: Unraveling the Complexities of Ambiguous Language and Humor was designed to teach individuals, age 10 through adulthood, to recognize and interpret ambiguous language, to identify and explain words and expressions that have both literal and nonliteral meanings, to detect and resolve incongruity in humor items, to recognize and explain particular elements of humor, and to recognize humor cues. This resource has the flexibility to teach these skills in a book format or a game format (using the 16" × 16" game mat provided).

Part I: Introduction covers such topics as the goals, target audience, and rationale for this resource; the use of contextual support and a cognitive-strategies approach for instruction; and the method for assessing comprehension of ambiguous language and humor. Part II: Activities presents seven units covering a variety of linguistic elements. The tasks include both traditional, academic-type items and humorous items. The activity pages may be reproduced and handed out or made into overheads and then conducted orally with individuals.

- Unit 1 deals with multiple-meanings words—both homographs and homophones.

- Unit 2 targets multiple-meaning phrases using items that delve into the meanings of idioms and proverbs.

- Unit 3 presents multiple-meaning sentences.

- Unit 4 explores meaning changes caused by sound (i.e., phoneme) changes.

- Unit 5 deals with understanding the multiple meanings that are caused by switching sounds or words.

- Unit 6 targets the effect of stress and juncture changes on the meaning of a message.

- Unit 7 provides challenge items—a mixture of tasks containing metaphors and similes, as well as a variety of verbal and visual humor items based on the manipulation of language.

Each unit includes background information, related research, and procedural information specific to the types of targets that are found within the unit. As a convenience, answer keys for the activities also are included at the end of each unit.

In addition to Parts I and II, there are five useful appendices. Appendix A is a reproducible recording form for assessing an individual's understanding of ambiguous language and humor. Appendix B is a convenient guide that lists the definitions of the idioms and proverbs used in the units (unless defined within the text of an activity) and other common idioms and proverbs.

Appendix C contains 150 reproducible game cards to be used with the provided game mat. (The game card tasks are similar in style and scope to the other items in this resource.) Appendix D supplies a reproducible template for creating additional game cards. Appendix E provides the answer key to the game card items in Appendix C.

Goals

As Far as Words Go provides the facilitator with numerous opportunities to help individuals address semantic, metalinguistic, and pragmatic skills that require strengthening. The activities offer a relaxed context for communication in which these and other language goals can be achieved:

Semantic Skills

- Providing two meanings for ambiguous words or phrases

- Recognizing and explaining the difference between the literal and figurative meanings of idioms

- Demonstrating an understanding of inferences in material that can have two interpretations

- Identifying humor that results from multiple-meaning words or phrases

Metalinguistic Skills

- Recognizing and describing how the manipulation of phonemes can create humor

- Identifying the sounds, words, or phrases that cause humor in language

- Recognizing stress and juncture changes that alter the meaning of a statement

- Integrating visually presented material, such as word puzzles, into a verbal framework

Pragmatic Skills

- Requesting additional information, clarification, or repetition of a message when necessary

- Acting appropriately as both a speaker and a listener during communication exchanges

- Using socially appropriate turn-taking behaviors

Target Audience

A wide range of individuals are likely to benefit from the activities in _As Far as Words Go._ The activities in both the book and game format were specifically designed for preadolescents, adolescents, and adults who:

- Have a language disorder or language-based learning disability

- Have a reading disability

- Are learning English as a foreign language

- Have incurred brain injuries

- Have a mild form of autism or a related disability

- Possess typical learning and achievement but want to improve their ability to understand ambiguous language and humor

The material in this resource may be too difficult for individuals who have severe cognitive deficits, such as those with moderate to profound degrees of cognitive disabilities or some forms of autism.

Facilitators who might use this resource include speech-language pathologists, special education teachers, learning disabilities specialists, general education teachers, remedial reading specialists, and teachers of English as a foreign language.

Background
Rationale

Ambiguous language occurs frequently in textbooks, magazines, newspapers, novels, television programs, and movies. Magazine advertisements and television and radio commercials rely on ambiguous material to capture our attention. For example, a magazine advertisement for a carpet-cleaning product shows a piece of chocolate cake that has fallen and stained a carpet. The advertisement reads, "To us this is a piece of cake." Researchers have shown that such examples of ambiguous language and humor are problematic for individuals with weak language skills (e.g., Abrahamsen and Sprouse, 1995; Larson and McKinley, 1995; Lloyd, 1994; Nelson, 1993; Nippold, 1991, 1998; Nippold and Rudzinski, 1993; Secord and Wiig, 1993; Spector, 1990, 1992, 1996). Understanding and use of these aspects of language are impeded by a limited vocabulary base, restrictive world knowledge, poor reading proficiency, weak analogical reasoning, and difficulty treating language metalinguistically (Milosky, 1990; Nippold, Allen, and Kirsch, 2001; Spector, 1990; van Kleeck, 1984). The extent to which any one of these factors affects the comprehension of ambiguous language and humor is not clear. It is likely that these factors interact with one another. Perhaps individuals with reduced language skills simply lack experience with the full range of nonliteral language used by their counterparts who have typical language skills. In any case, to have appropriate social interactions and academic achievement, and to be truly literate, one must be able to understand ambiguous language and humor (Spector, 1997). The degree to which ambiguous language and humor pervade our everyday lives, both orally and in text, emphasizes the need for children and adults to be able to interpret such items. Furthermore, an inability to understand linguistic ambiguities and humor may lead to:

- Feelings of inadequacy in understanding what others seem to understand

- Embarrassment

- Reduced academic performance

- Literacy challenges

- Stifled social interactions, which may lead to a sense of isolation

- Lack of confidence about participating in verbal interactions in school, in extracurricular activities, at home, or on the job

- Feeling powerless in coping with school, social, or job-related situations

- Loss of the pleasure found in the many forms of humor and wordplay based on linguistic ambiguities

As Far as Words Go explores various aspects of ambiguous language and humor and offers a variety of intervention activities that will improve an individual's ability to understand and use figurative language.

Ambiguous Language and the Linguistic Elements of Humor

Ambiguous language refers to a message that can be interpreted in two or more ways; *humor* is a message that contains an amusing quality. Language can be ambiguous, humorous, or both at the same time. Everyday spontaneous conversations and school language are replete with ambiguous language and humor. One's ability to determine the appropriate interpretation of ambiguities and humor is affected by many factors, such as the linguistic and social context; the individual's familiarity with the linguistic elements; and whether the material is oral, written, or both.

As shown in Table 1 (see page 8), there are 10 linguistic elements of humor. One of these elements is lexical (i.e., semantic) items, 3 of the elements involve humor at the phonological level, 4 include items at the morphological level, and 2 include humor at the syntactic level. The most popular kinds of humor for older children, adolescents, and adults are based on a combination of the lexical (i.e., semantic), phonological, and syntactic elements (Spector, 1990). Therefore, humor based on the morphological elements is not included in the activities in _As Far as Words Go_.

Of the 6 linguistic humor elements described and targeted in this resource (i.e., in the first six units), 4 are based on ambiguities (i.e., multiple-meaning words, multiple-meaning phrases, multiple-meaning sentences, and stress and juncture changes) and 2 are based on humor that results from factors other than ambiguities (i.e., sound changes and switching sounds or words). The following are descriptions of these 6 linguistic humor elements:

Multiple-Meaning Words—Sometimes a single word in a message can be the source of ambiguity. For example, _great_ and _grate_ sound the same but are spelled differently. And just as _great_ can be interpreted in many ways (for example, one can have a _great_ number of things, King Kong was a _great_ ape, your grandmother's mother is your _great_-grandmother, Nobel prize winners are considered _great_ men and women, and one can look _great)_, so can _grate_ (for example, one can _grate_ potatoes to make potato pancakes, a shrill voice can _grate_ on a listener's nerves, and wood can be placed on a fireplace _grate)_. Humor of this type is a result of a _lexical_ linguistic element (i.e., lexical element I in Table 1).

Multiple-Meaning Phrases—Phrases with multiple meanings can be ambiguous, humorous, or both. Typically, multiple-meaning phrases are idioms. Phrases with multiple meanings can often be interpreted either literally or figuratively. For example, the phrase _butter up_ could literally mean "to spread butter over something" or figuratively mean "to flatter or compliment another person in order to win his or her favor." Humorous multiple-meaning phrases are a result of a _phrase structure_ linguistic element (i.e., syntactic element A in Table 1).

Multiple-Meaning Sentences—Multiple-meaning sentences can create ambiguity, humor, or both. For example, the sentence _Peter gave me a hand_ can be taken literally to mean "Peter gave me a hand" (e.g., a plaster hand from a mannequin) or figuratively in two ways—"Peter helped me" or "Peter applauded for me." A sentence such as a newspaper headline that reads _Dawson Gets Nine Months in Violin Case_ is also open to dual interpretation. It could mean "Dawson has to go to prison for nine months as a result of a legal case that involves a violin" or "Dawson will have to spend nine months in a case made to hold a violin." Humor of this type is a result of _transformational ambiguity_ (i.e., syntactic element B in Table 1).

Table 1   **Linguistic Humor Elements**

Type of Element	Basis of Humor	Example
I. Lexical	The ambiguity of a word.	"Janitors' union calls for *sweeping reform*."
II. Phonological A. Minimal pairs	Involves the difference of one phoneme.	"The inventors of the rocket went out to *launch*."
B. Metathesis	Sound reversal.	Usher in a movie theater: "Let me *sew* you to your *sheet*."
	Word reversal.	"What's the difference between a cat and a comma?" "A cat has *claws* at the end of its *paws*, and a comma is a *pause* at the end of a *clause*."
C. Stress/Juncture	The placement of stress changes the meaning.	"What would you have if everyone in the country drove a pink cadillac?" "A pink *car nation*."
III. Morphological A. Irregular morphology	Exploiting a misinterpretation of a grammatical form.	Sign in pottery shop: *"Feats of clay."*
B. Morphological analysis	One morpheme is extracted from a word and treated as if it were an independent word that it is homophonous with.	"I went to Ireland to get an emerald, but all I got was a *shamrock*."
C. Exploitation of bound morphemes	A bound morpheme is deliberately confused with an independent word or otherwise exploited.	"I must say, you're looking *couth*, *kempt*, and *sheveled* today."
D. Pseudomorphology	An independent word is deliberately confused with a phonological sequence from another, larger word, but the sequence is not really a morpheme of the larger word.	"What pet makes the best music?" "A trum*pet*."
IV. Syntactic A. Phrase structure	A given surface sequence of words has more than one syntactic analysis.	"When the first diet club was formed, it was a *losing proposition*."
B. Transformational ambiguity	Two different underlying structures have an identical surface form as a result of their respective syntactic derivations.	**Julie:** Do you realize it takes three sheep to make one sweater? **Bill:** I didn't even know that sheep could knit.

From "Linguistic Humor Comprehension of Normal and Language-Impaired Adolescents," by C.C. Spector, 1990, *Journal of Speech and Hearing Disorders, 55*, p. 534. © 1990 by the American Speech-Language-Hearing Association. Reprinted with permission.

Multiple-meaning words, phrases, or sentences may become ambiguous without the visual support offered by written text. Spelling, at times, provides clarifying information and helps support the appropriate interpretation. For example, consider the statements _She had some time_ versus _She had some thyme._ The ambiguity can be removed with the support of the visual cue.

Sound Changes—Humor is frequently based on the manipulation of phonemes within a word or statement (Green and Pepicello, 1978; Pepicello, 1980; Spector, 1990, 1997). For example, the statement _After reading a book she didn't like, the critic said, "This book should be on the bestsmeller list"_ is humorous because of the addition of /m/ to change the word _bestseller_ to _bestsmeller._ The linguistic element of _minimal pairs_ explains this type of humor (i.e., phonological element A in Table 1).

Switching Sounds or Words—Humor can also be caused by the intentional or accidental transposition of sounds or words within a statement. For example, in the statement _One frog said to another, "Time sure is fun when you're having flies,"_ the humor is a result of the words _fun_ and _flies_ being switched (and the addition of _is_). _Metathesis_ is the linguistic element responsible for this type of humor (i.e., phonological element B in Table 1).

Stress and Juncture Changes—Punctuation (which can indicate stress, intonation, and juncture) also helps provide information necessary for proper interpretation of a potentially ambiguous or humorous statement. For example, a major difference in meaning can be caused by adding a comma (e.g., _Jump over, Sally_ versus _Jump over Sally_) or by adding a comma and changing the placement of a comma (e.g., _Woman without her man, is nothing_ versus _Woman, without her, man is nothing_). These types of alterations can result in a simple ambiguity or they can create humor. Stress and juncture humor is caused by a _phonological_ linguistic element (i.e., phonological element C in Table 1).

Facilitating the Acquisition of Ambiguous Language and Humor

A wide range of metacognitive, metapragmatic, and metalinguistic skills (i.e., skills affecting the ability to "know that you know") are required for an individual to understand and use ambiguous language and humor. For example, as Spector (1997) pointed out, to truly understand and use such elements, a person must be able to:

- Detect the presence of ambiguous material

- Recognize ambiguous material from stored memory

- Evoke new and different meanings in words, phrases, and sentences

- Define words

- Interpret ambiguous information literally and figuratively

- Analyze and integrate syntactic information

- Explain multiple meanings

- Put into words what is known implicitly

- Generalize meaning from use in other contexts

- Infer meaning

- Perceive and use paralinguistic cues (i.e., vocal intensity, stress, and intonation)

- Paraphrase to clarify meaning

- Segment and redefine a phonological string

- Revise an utterance to fulfill a listener's needs

- Perceive shifts in perspective

- Monitor one's own utterances

- Recognize a listener's inability to understand an utterance

- Provide appropriate repairs to communication breakdowns

Metacognitive abilities such as attending, organizing, remembering, and problem solving affect the development of metalinguistic skills. Metapragmatic abilities for activities such as requesting information or revising an utterance also affect the development of metacognitive and metalinguistic skills. No clear-cut lines of distinction can be drawn among these domains of awareness. Each will have some impact on the others.

Given that ambiguous language and humor are so prevalent in our everyday lives, individuals with language-learning disorders and individuals who are learning English as a foreign language may need to be shown how to abstract meaning from context. This can be accomplished through repeated exposure to ambiguous language and humor accompanied by instructional support and facilitation (Nelson, 1993; Spector, 1992; Wiig and Wiig, 1999). Possible deficits in understanding nonliteral language must be given serious consideration when planning intervention for older children, adolescents, and adults. Providing contextual support, using a cognitive-strategies approach, and using explanation tasks can facilitate the acquisition of figurative language.

Contextual Support

Individuals who need to improve their understanding of ambiguous language and humor most likely have already been exposed to such language in their natural environment. Their difficulty in mastering these aspects of language on their own indicates that a facilitator is needed to provide additional opportunities and structure for learning them (Brown, Anderson, Shillcock, and Yule, 1984; Wiig and Wiig, 1999). Individuals who have problems understanding abstract or ambiguous language because they have poor metalinguistic awareness also are likely to achieve greater success by working with a facilitator than they would by working on their own.

The more frequently an ambiguous or humorous statement is heard in spontaneous conversation, the more familiar it will become. However, familiarity alone does not ensure that one can understand the meaning of such a statement. Contextual support for the appropriate interpretation is also essential. Further, certain ambiguous utterances may be used by some groups and not by others. Therefore, one's degree of familiarity with any particular ambiguous statement also can depend on the statement's usage by individuals in a particular age range, cultural group, or geographic location.

The use of contrived materials (e.g., activity sheets and games) with appropriate, well-developed contextual support appears to be a logical solution. Basic skills needed for understanding ambiguous language and humor can be established through activities developed specifically for that purpose. Larson and McKinley (1995) suggested that such materials and activities be developed along a continuum that eventually leads to understanding in natural settings (i.e., generalization).

For academic-type tasks, contextual support can be manipulated to provide the degree of support necessary for comprehension. Take this story for example:

Jane came home after midnight even though she had a 10PM curfew. This was the third time she came home late this month, and she knew her parents would be very angry. She was sure that her father would hit the roof.

The context of this story not only supports the idiom *hit the roof*, it also defines it ("to become very angry"). A less-supportive context would be:

Jane was worried that her father would hit the roof when she got home.

This statement provides little contextual support. An individual would need to stretch his or her inferencing skills to connect the word *worried* to the idiom *hit the roof* in order to interpret its meaning.

Context clues available for jokes, riddles, signs, advertisements, and so forth cannot be manipulated as easily. The clues are inherent to the items. Some provide clues that support literal interpretations, some provide clues that support figurative interpretations, and some provide clues that support both literal and figurative interpretations.

At first, a great deal of contextual support will be needed to lead an individual to the correct interpretation of an ambiguous or humorous message. Eventually, less and less contextual support will be needed as an individual becomes more adept at using all available linguistic and nonlinguistic cues.

A Cognitive-Strategies Approach

As Far as Words Go uses a cognitive-strategies approach suggested by Seidenberg (1988) to address deficits in the comprehension of linguistic-based humor, much of which is based on figurative language and other ambiguities. The goals of this approach are to:

- Improve the individual's awareness of the demands of the task

- Help the individual find the relevant strategy

- Describe the strategy to the individual

- Teach the individual how to apply a relevant strategy in controlled practice materials

The following principles of a cognitive-strategies approach are enumerated and described in *Saying One Thing, Meaning Another* (Spector, 1997). Adhering to these principles will enable professionals to get the most beneficial results from their efforts to facilitate language learning.

- Consider the individual's current level of development or functioning.

- Adjust assistance to fit the needs of the individual, taking interests and past experiences into account.

- Assist the individual in learning the process of identifying the steps in an activity.

- Mediate an activity's level of difficulty so that the individual can realize greater levels of competency without being overwhelmed.

- Assist the individual in expanding (or regaining) world knowledge.

- Assist the individual in developing pragmatic skills, such as knowing "when to say what."

- Assist the individual in developing problem-solving procedures.

- Promote the individual's ability to make inferences.

- Present materials in varying formats that are consistent with the individual's interests.

- Assist the individual in developing (or regaining) reasoning skills.

- Provide naturalistic contexts whenever possible.

- Assist in the development of repair strategies when there is a miscommunication of meaning.

Implementing this cognitive-strategies approach is predicated on the individual having, or being able to attain, an adequate level of metalinguistic awareness. *Metalinguistic awareness,* as described by van Kleeck (1984), is the ability to reflect on language as an entity and the ability to compartmentalize language into its linguistic units. The development of metalinguistic skills generally occurs between 7 and 12 years of age with the advent of concrete operational thinking (Piaget, 1954). However, many children and adolescents with impaired language abilities have not adequately developed these skills, and in individuals who have sustained head trauma, had a cerebrovascular accident, or incurred some other neurological impairment, these skills may become weakened.

The activities in *As Far as Words Go* foster the development of metalinguistic skills such as evoking new and different meanings of words and phrases, determining the nature of phonologically based sound differences, segmenting and redefining phonological strings, interpreting words and phrases literally and figuratively, integrating contextual information, and putting into words what is known implicitly.

Using Explanation Tasks

Explanation tasks are usually more difficult than multiple- or forced-choice formats and may, therefore, underestimate one's level of understanding in assessment procedures (Nippold et al., 2001; Nippold and Rudzinski, 1993). Multiple- or forced-choice formats allow the individual to show comprehension in a passive manner. However, there are several reasons for using explanation tasks in intervention activities like those found in this resource.

- Explanation tasks are a more rigorous way of showing comprehension of ambiguous language and humor because they require a greater depth of knowledge. To provide explanations, an individual must develop the metalinguistic skills needed for active (rather than passive) understanding and for communicating meaning in a clear manner. According to Vygotsky's (1962) theory, if these skills are perceived as weak, it is possible to facilitate their development.

- Explanations often are required in real-life situations; multiple choices are rarely offered. Gaining experience with explanation tasks involving ambiguous language and humor can be a useful method of improving an individual's ability to provide explanations in other language areas.

- The nature of some items do not lend themselves to multiple-choice formats. Stress and juncture items, for example, are based on an individual's ability to select a phonological string and resegment it to form a new meaning. A multiple-choice format would compromise the selection procedure.

- Explanations frequently are needed in academic subjects. Although explanations may underestimate passive understanding, they allow facilitators to gain insight into qualitative changes as the individual continues to work on a specific language task. Facilitators then have the opportunity to examine the individual's explanation and determine what is needed for him or her to gain a true understanding of the specific task.

Assessing Comprehension of Ambiguous Language and Humor

Standardized measures for assessing comprehension of all the linguistic elements in this resource do not exist. However, by using a variety of items from the first six units of *As Far as Words Go*, an individual's understanding of ambiguous language and humor can be informally measured before and after he or she participates in the activities.

Appendix A contains a reproducible form for recording the informal assessment results of an individual's comprehension of each type of linguistic humor element targeted in *As Far as Words Go*. Given that each linguistic humor element may have items with a different number of possible responses, it is best to show the number of correct responses in relation to the number of possible responses for each item.

For example, if a multiple-meaning words item has four separate questions and the individual gets one correct, write 1/4 in one of the small rectangular boxes across from the Multiple-Meaning Words heading. Up to three different items can be scored for each type of linguistic humor element (i.e., three Multiple-Meaning Words items, three Multiple-Meaning Phrases items, etc.). A subtotal for each of the six linguistic humor elements can also be derived and placed in the larger squares next to the smaller rectangular boxes. In addition, cumulative preintervention and postintervention scores can be derived and indicated in the spaces at the bottom of the form. This type of scoring can be used for both preintervention assessment and posttesting. A completed recording form is shown in Figure 1.

Use the Comments area at the bottom of the form to indicate any special notes or unusual circumstances related to either the preintervention or postintervention assessment procedures

Figure 1   *Recording Form* Example

Recording Form NAME: _Jimmy K._

PreTest Date: _9/21/01_   Posttest Date: _3/16/02_

TASK TYPE	PREINTERVENTION PERFORMANCE (# OF CORRECT RESPONSES / # OF TASKS)		POSTINTERVENTION PERFORMANCE (# OF CORRECT RESPONSES / # OF TASKS)	
MULTIPLE-MEANING WORDS	2 / 4 1 / 4 2 / 4	5 / 12	3 / 4 4 / 4 3 / 4	10 / 12
MULTIPLE-MEANING PHRASES	0 / 4 1 / 3 1 / 4	2 / 11	2 / 4 3 / 3 2 / 2	7 / 9
MULTIPLE-MEANING SENTENCES	3 / 4 0 / 3 0 / 4	3 / 11	4 / 4 2 / 4 2 / 3	8 / 11
SOUND CHANGES	0 / 4 1 / 4 2 / 4	3 / 12	4 / 4 3 / 4 4 / 4	11 / 12
SWITCHING SOUNDS OR WORDS	2 / 2 1 / 3 1 / 4	4 / 9	3 / 3 2 / 3 3 / 4	8 / 10
STRESS AND PAUSING CHANGES	2 / 4 0 / 3 1 / 4	3 / 11	3 / 4 3 / 3 3 / 4	9 / 11
TOTALS	■	20 / 66	■	53 / 65

COMMENTS:

Pretest: Jimmy asked many questions and attempted to gain a great deal of assistance during all tasks.

Posttest: Jimmy was confident and worked independently to complete tasks.

(e.g., if a student was extraordinarily tired or responded to all items very quickly). Date each assessment session in the space provided at the top of the form, and keep the completed form in the individual's file or portfolio.

Using *As Far as Words Go*

Each of the first six units in *As Far as Words Go* present activities addressing a single linguistic humor element (e.g., multiple-meaning words). The seventh unit is a mixture of challenging items across all elements, as well as other types of items that are based on linguistic manipulation. All the activities are appropriate for one-to-one or group interaction. While one-to-one interaction may focus more on the needs of an individual, working with groups offers increased opportunities for brainstorming and social interaction.

Organization of the Units

In the seven units of *As Far as Words Go,* the activity pages are grouped by the types of ambiguities or humor they address. All seven units include activities that have humorous elements. Three of these units also include activities that are not humor based.

Humorous Language

As Far as Words Go contains activities based on six linguistic elements of humor (see Table 1, page 8). For the purposes of this resource, the six linguistic humor elements—lexical items, phrase structure, transformational ambiguity, minimal pairs, metathesis, and stress and juncture changes—are delineated in the following activity units:

Multiple-Meaning Words (lexical items)—Unit 1 includes homograph and homophone items that result in humor, such as:

> Q. What do you call a conference of mummies?

> A. A wrap session.

>> a. Which word in the answer is used to make this joke funny?

>> b. What does it mean the way it is spelled above?

>> c. How else can it be spelled and what would it mean?

>> d. Which words or phrases give you a clue to each meaning?

Multiple-Meaning Phrases (phrase structure)—Phrases that can have two or more interpretations are targeted in Unit 2 through items such as:

> Q. How does a puppet get into show business?
> A. He has someone pull a few strings for him.

>> a. Which phrase in the answer can have two meanings?

>> b. What does it mean here?

>> c. What else can it mean?

>> d. Which words or phrases in the question give you clues to one of the meanings?

Multiple-Meaning Sentences (transformational ambiguity)—In Unit 3, sentences with multiple meanings form the basis for items such as:

Sign in a nursery: "All Babies Are Subject to Change without Notice"

> *a. Explain the two meanings of this sign.*
>
> *b. Which words or phrases give you a clue to the intended meaning of the sign?*

Sound Changes (minimal pairs)—Humor that is caused by changes in individual sounds in words are the focus of Unit 4's activities. These activity types fall into four categories—adding a phoneme, changing a consonant phoneme, changing a vowel phoneme, and taking away a phoneme. The following is an example of one of these activities:

There's a scale over there. Go weigh!

> *a. Which word makes this joke funny?*
>
> *b. What do you think the real word is?*
>
> *c. Which words or phrases give you a clue to why the funny word is used?*
>
> *d. Explain why the funny word is used.*

Switching Sounds or Words (metathesis)—Sound or word transpositions that create humor are targeted in the Unit 5 activities. For example:

Usher in a darkened movie theater: "Let me sew you to your sheet."

> *a. Which sounds in this joke are switched?*
>
> *b. What does the usher mean to say?*
>
> *c. Which words or phrases give you a clue to what the usher means?*
>
> *d. Why are the sounds switched in this way?*

Stress and Juncture Changes—Alterations to the stress and/or juncture of a statement resulting in humor is the focus of Unit 6's activities. (NOTE: The simpler label of *pausing*, rather than *juncture*, is used to label these types of tasks within the unit.) An example of such an activity is:

Bestseller: Will He or Won't He?
> *by Mae B. Sew*

> *a. What funny meaning can the author's name have?*
>
> *b. Which words or phrases give you a clue to the funny meaning?*

Academic-Type Ambiguities

Unit 1: Multiple-Meaning Words, Unit 2: Multiple-Meaning Phrases, and Unit 7: Challenge Activities also contain some academic-type activities that are not humor based, such as the following:

Multiple-Meaning Words—Unit 1 includes homograph items in which individuals are asked to provide two or more definitions for a word that sounds the same and is spelled the same as another word but has multiple meanings. For example:

Write at least two sentences that show different meanings for the word slip.

Another type of homograph activity instructs individuals to provide definitions for each pronunciation of a word that is spelled the same as another word but has a different meaning and a different pronunciation. For example:

present—Sue was selected to **present** *the* **present** *to Tom.*

    a. present:

    b. present:

Homophone pairs in which individuals are asked to make a sentence incorporating both members of the pair are also included in Unit 1. For example:

Write one sentence that contains the words deer/dear.

Multiple-Meaning Phrases—Finding like-meaning idioms and defining proverbs are included as academic-type tasks in Unit 2. For example:

Bury the hatchet *means "to try to make peace." What means the same as* bury the hatchet?

    a. riding for a fall   b. face the music   c. hold out an olive branch

Challenge Activities—In this unit, academic-type items ask individuals to select the appropriate meanings of metaphors and similes. For example:

    1. Joe was like a fish out of water.

        a. What do you think this simile means?

          • *Joe was flopping around.*
          • *Joe was all dry.*
          • *Joe was feeling awkward and uncomfortable.*

        b. Why might someone act like a fish out of water?

Presenting the Activities

Facilitator pages, which precede the activities in each unit, include helpful background information, presentation suggestions, and one or more examples. Present the example items for teaching and discussion before individual or group work on each unit.

Each type of activity within a unit (except Unit 7) contains an _Introductory Activity Page_ and two or more corresponding activity pages. The _Introductory Activity Page_ provides definitions, detailed information regarding the ambiguous language and humor being targeted, suggestions for interpreting the targeted language forms, one or more completed items to review, and one or more items to complete together. These pages are intended to be discussed orally.

An attempt was made to hierarchically arrange the items within each of the first six units. Given the wide range of differences between individuals' world knowledge, vocabulary base, familiarity with figurative expressions, ability to use contextual clues, and so forth, the resulting hierarchy will not necessarily be applicable for all individuals. Therefore, use discretion when choosing appropriate activity pages for individuals.

The following suggests an effective strategy for presenting the activity pages.

1. Based on assessment results, determine an individual's goals and select a corresponding activity (e.g., Unit 1, Activity 1: Developing Sentences for Words with Multiple Meanings).

2. Read through the facilitator information provided at the beginning of the unit you have selected.

3. Duplicate the _Introductory Activity Page_ and one or more corresponding activity pages for the selected target (e.g., pages 36–39 when targeting Unit 1, Activity 1 for the first time).

   NOTE: If the _Introductory Activity Page_ for a particular skill was used in a previous session with an individual or a group, it does not have to be used during a subsequent session targeting the same skill. Instead, duplicate one or more corresponding activity pages for use. However, it may also be beneficial to have a completed copy of that activity's introductory page on hand as a reference during the session. Also note that _Introductory Activity Pages_ do not exist for Unit 7: Challenge Activities.

4. Distribute and discuss the selected _Introductory Activity Page_ (or review the one that was completed during a previous session). Also consider bringing in and discussing additional

task examples, like those provided in the unit's facilitator pages.

> NOTE: When working with a group, consider making overhead transparencies to use during the activity rather than, or in addition to, using handouts.

5. Read the activity directions and work together to complete the introductory example items and discuss responses. Facilitate a discussion about any troublesome items. The decision of whether to conduct an activity orally or to have individuals read and complete an activity on their own should be based on what would be most beneficial for each individual. Consider goals, reading skills, visual acuity, level of independence, and so forth. When possible, it is best for individuals to see each item as well as hear it read aloud.

> NOTE: Some tasks will require written presentation. For example, for the following item to be humorous, the visual cue of spelling *time* as *thyme* is essential:

> *Q. Why did the cook hurry to the herb garden?*

> *A. He didn't have much thyme.*

Also decide whether responses to the remaining stimulus items will be written or oral. Again, this decision should be made on an individual basis. The method of activity presentation—on paper, on an overhead projector, or both—also will affect this decision. If desired, compare each individual's responses with those in the answer key. (Use Appendix B: Definitions of Idioms and Proverbs, if necessary, when working on items containing idioms or proverbs.)

6. Collect completed activity pages in a file or portfolio for each individual, or encourage individuals to take their pages home to share with a family member or friend.

Using the Game Format

A 16" × 16" game mat is included with this book. The colored spaces on the mat represent the different elements of ambiguous language and humor targeted in the seven units of the book. The following color key for the five decks is provided on the game mat.

> Yellow=Multiple-meaning words
>
> Green=Multiple-meaning phrases
>
> Red=Multiple-meaning sentences, switching sounds or words, and stress and pausing changes
>
> Orange=Sound changes
>
> Blue=Challenge activities

Appendix C contains 150 game cards (30 cards for each deck) for use with the game mat. The items on the game cards are similar to those provided on the activity pages of the resource. Additional types of items are included in the Challenge Activities deck. The red deck contains items for three linguistic elements—multiple-meaning sentences, switching sounds or word, and stress and pausing changes. Each of these elements is represented by relatively few items, thus they were combined to form one deck.

Setting Up

Use the following procedure to prepare for game play:

1. Duplicate each page from Appendix C onto the specified color of paper (e.g., copy the multiple-meaning words pages onto yellow paper). The recommended color for each card deck is indicated at the top of each page in Appendix C. For added durability, use heavy-stock paper or consider laminating the cards.

   > NOTE: If colored paper is not available, copy the pages onto white heavy-stock paper and use magic markers, crayons, or colored dot stickers to color-code the back side of each card prior to laminating the pages and cutting the cards apart.

   If during later rounds of play you need additional game cards, feel free to create them using items from the activity pages in the book. Simply duplicate Appendix D as often as needed and write the additional items on the Game Card Template. (Be sure to color-code these cards based on the types of ambiguous language and humor targeted.)

2. Cut the pages along dotted lines to create cards.

3. Sort the cards by color into decks. (Consider storing the decks in plastic zipper bags.)

4. Collect two to six (depending on the number of players) tokens, coins, colored paper clips, marker caps, or colored scraps of paper to use as game pawns.

Playing the Game

The *As Far as Words Go* game can be played by 2 to 6 people at a time. When working with a single individual, the facilitator should become a player in order to use the game format. Ideally, the game activity should be used after an individual has had at least some exposure to the activities provided in the book. The following game play is recommended:

1. Set out the game mat and place the card decks around the mat so that they can be reached by all players. Each player should choose one of the six "ladders" on the game mat to use during a round of play. Suggest that each player sit near his or her ladder.

2. Have each player choose a game pawn and place it on the Start spot of his or her ladder.

3. Designate a player to be first.

4. The starting player should move his or her game pawn to the first colored spot on his or her ladder. He or she should then select the top card from that deck and read it aloud.

   > NOTES: Either the player or the facilitator can read the card, depending on the player's reading skills. When the facilitator is also the reader, he or she should be sure to show the card to the player so that the visual cues are related. The card should be shown to all players when a visual representation is included.
   >
   > There are usually several questions on each card. Decide whether the player must respond to all or only some of the questions (e.g., you can have players skip explanation-task questions if they appear to be too difficult for the player).
   >
   > Several game cards are marked with a star (★). These items are judged to be more challenging than other cards in the same deck. When players answer one of these cards correctly, they should move forward two spaces on their ladders.
   >
   > Several game cards are marked with a square (■). To add variation to the game, a player who selects one of these cards may choose to respond to the item or have the facilitator respond (individuals love to put the facilitator "on the spot"). After the correct responses have been discussed, the player who selected the card is the one who gets to move forward.

5. Judge and discuss the appropriateness of the player's response. If desired, have other players give their input regarding the response. Although the answer key in Appendix E provides a list of possible correct responses for the game card items from Appendix C, judging the correctness of the answers is left to the discretion of the facilitator. If responses are judged to be acceptable, the player should move his or her game pawn up the ladder to the next colored space. If responses are judged to be incorrect, the player should remain on the space

and attempt an item from the same color deck on his or her next turn. (As an alternative, have players move ahead regardless of the correctness of a response, as long as the correct responses have been discussed.)

> NOTE: When moving up the ladder, there are two times when a player must choose between two different colored spaces (i.e., at the fourth and seventh "steps"). Call the player's attention to the color key on the board to help him or her decide which color space would be preferred.

6. Play then moves clockwise to the next player.

7. When a player reaches the Final Challenge space, a card from the Challenge Activities deck (i.e., the blue deck) is read. The first player or players to climb their ladder and correctly respond to a Challenge Activity card win. Be sure to provide players with an equal number of turns before declaring a single player the winner. If there is insufficient time to finish the game, the player or players who are closest to the Final Challenge space can be declared the winners.

Using the Game in a Classroom Setting

For larger groups, use the five game card decks without the game mat. Simply divide the group into two or more teams. Place five colored tokens (yellow, green, red, orange, and blue) into a nontransparent container. Without looking, the teams should take turns selecting a token and responding to an item on a card of the same color as the chosen token. As the teams take turns, keep a tally of correct responses. The team with the most correct responses after a predetermined number of turns can be declared the winner.

> NOTE: When teams respond to a card marked with a star (★), they should earn two points. When presented with a card marked with a square (■), the team can earn one point by responding or by asking the facilitator to respond to the item.

Promoting Generalization of Skills

Generalization of the skills targeted in *As Far as Words Go* is likely to increase because of the cognitive-strategies approach used throughout the activities. However, there are extension activities and facilitator techniques that can add to the likelihood that strategies for understanding and using ambiguous language and humor will transfer to other situations and settings.

Extension Activities

The following five activities are offered as additional ways for helping individuals understand and use multiple-meaning words, multiple-meaning phrases, multiple-meaning sentences, sound changes, sound or word switching, and stress and juncture changes.

1. Have individuals scan a newspaper (the sports section is especially rich in ambiguous material) or magazine and underline or circle elements of ambiguous language. Discuss the highlighted elements as they relate to the context of the reading material. Consider using the structured explanation-task format that is used throughout the activity pages and game cards in this resource to discuss the new examples found in the newspaper or magazine.

2. Direct individuals to write down confusing ambiguous messages as they encounter them. Sources for these messages could be spontaneous conversations, classroom discussions, movies, television programs, or written materials. Routinely discuss these messages and encourage individuals to use other resources (e.g., dictionary or thesaurus) to figure out unclear statements.

3. Ask individuals to examine cartoons and comic strips for examples of humor that stem from any of the language forms discussed in this resource. Collect these examples in a book and use them as a basis for recurring discussions.

4. Present segments of movies, television programs, or television commercials on videotape. Strategically select samples that demonstrate intentionally ambiguous language or humor based on the linguistic humor elements in Table 1 (see page 8). Hold a discussion to help individuals recognize and understand the ambiguities or humorous qualities captured in the video clips.

5. Encourage individuals to collect samples of ambiguous language and humor from textbooks, store signs, billboards, bumper stickers, tee shirts, and so on. These examples can then be discussed and interpreted appropriately using the cognitive-strategies approach and the explanation tasks used throughout *As Far as Words Go*.

Facilitator Techniques

In addition to the extension activities, facilitators can use the following techniques for promoting acquisition of skills and generalization of new skills to other situations and settings.

Using Verbal Mediation

Many individuals are likely to have difficulty with some of the items in this book. Offer ongoing verbal mediation, especially when presenting the *Introductory Activity Pages* and practice items. Such types of verbal mediation might include, but should not be limited to, the following:

- Elicit understanding from the individual by asking guiding questions that help reframe and refine the individual's response.

- Supply extra information, such as vocabulary definitions.

- Provide some aspect of world knowledge.

- Point out and discuss context clues.

- Even if the individual provides a correct response to an item, promote divergent thinking by asking further process-oriented questions, such as "How did you know which one to select?" "Why is that choice better than the others?" "What did you do to solve this item?" and "Is there another way to look at the item?"

- Ask for "bridging" information from the individual. For example, ask "Can you think of another context in which you might use the same kind of thinking?"

Always discuss all responses to the questions that follow each item so that a correct pattern of response is set. Continue to offer verbal mediation whenever necessary.

Brainstorming

Learning to understand ambiguous language and humor is a form of problem solving. Brainstorming with individuals is one way of finding correct responses when items are missed. When brainstorming is used, acknowledge all responses provided without making judgments regarding quality or correctness. This technique promotes the active involvement of each individual when working with a group. Encourage ongoing discussion about questions and responses. Perhaps display a list of responses that were generated during brainstorming and review each to determine correct responses.

Thinking Aloud

Have individuals think aloud when attempting to figure out problematic items. Encourage individuals to verbalize their thoughts as they work through a task. Model this technique by saying things like:

- "I remember that the word *rock* can have several meanings. I need to figure out what it means in this sentence."

- "Oh, I see! I could pronounce the word by saying 'tennis' or I could say 'ten is.'"

- "I know the word *fly* can mean the insect or the action. I need to figure out what it means in this sentence."

- "I need to think about both meanings of that sentence."

- "If I say 'lunch time,' the sentence doesn't seem funny. If I change the vowel sound and say 'launch time,' the joke is funny to me."

- "Changing the stress and adding a pause changes the meaning of the words."

- "I need to remember to try different stress and pausing to see if I can change the meaning of the sentence to make it funny."

Explaining Unfamiliar Vocabulary

Individuals' performance can be adversely affected by their inability to understand some of the vocabulary in the activity items. Vocabulary that is problematic or new should be discussed as it appears. If necessary, provide definitions or encourage individuals to refer to dictionaries and other reference sources. Also encourage individuals to keep notes regarding meanings of new or problematic terms.

Assessing World Knowledge

Before beginning any activity, preview the activity pages or game cards looking for aspects of world knowledge that, in your judgment, may be unknown to the individual. Preteach or discuss this information when appropriate. Discussing possibly unknown or sophisticated aspects of world knowledge ensures better understanding of the activity items. For example:

Q. What do you get if a child stands under a falling piano?

A. A flat minor.

A discussion of musical terminology would support comprehension of this item. If such discussions are not appropriate or helpful, skipping over or setting aside such items is recommended.

Encouraging Discourse Skills

Encourage and facilitate ongoing discussions about the activity items. These discussions will provide opportunities for individuals to develop an awareness of the visual and verbal cues that signal ambiguities and humor, as well as opportunities to practice conversational skills.

The following outcomes can result when facilitator techniques are used:

- Alternate responses can be considered.

- Points of confusion can be identified.

- Context clues can be recognized and discussed.

- Analogies can be drawn to what is already known.

- Repair strategies can be used when there is a failure to comprehend.

- Unknown vocabulary can be defined.

- Additional, helpful information (i.e., clues) is provided.

- Understanding and use of vocabulary and concepts is heightened.

- Awareness of alternate settings and situations for applying new skills can be gained.

Enjoy the activities provided within _As Far as Words Go._ Most of all, help individuals see the humor and pleasure that can be found through the manipulation of linguistic elements of the English language.

Part II
ACTiViTY UNiTS

Unit 1:
Multiple-Meaning Words

Facilitator Information

Background

Words with multiple meanings appear to be easier to understand than other types of linguistic ambiguities (i.e., sentences with two meanings, phrases with multiple meanings, and ambiguities caused by changes in stress and juncture) (Spector, 1990). It is necessary for individuals to understand and manipulate words with multiple meanings before they can understand other types of figurative language, such as idioms and proverbs (Wiig and Semel, 1984).

The ability to define words and their multiple meanings is important because it is closely associated with academic achievement, reading proficiency, verbal ability, and intellectual performance in school-age children and adolescents (Nippold, Allen, and Kirsch, 2001; Snow, Cancini, Gonzalez, and Shriberg, 1989; Watson, 1985). The ability to define is implicit in grasping a word's multiple meanings.

The ability to resolve ambiguities involving multiple-meaning words begins when children reach the stage of cognitive development Piaget (1954) called *concrete operational thinking*. This occurs between 7 and 12 years of age. The ability to define words continues to develop into adulthood (Nippold, Hegel, Sohlberg, and Schwarz, 1999).

The Activities in This Unit

These activities provide opportunities for individuals to examine, learn, and use the following types of multiple-meaning words:

1. *Homographs* (first type)—where a target word sounds the same and is spelled the same as another word but has a different meaning (e.g., *rock, fly*).

2. *Homographs* (second type)—where a target word is spelled the same as another word but has a different meaning and a different pronunciation (e.g., *record, bass*).

3. *Homophones*—where a target word sounds the same as another word but has a different meaning and a different spelling (e.g., *reel/real, bare/bear*).

The activity types are organized as follows:

Activity 1—Each of the items contain a homograph of the first type, where the given word has more than one meaning but is spelled and pronounced the same way. Some of the words have several different meanings. Individuals are asked to see how many different sentences they can create that show different meanings for the given words.

Activity 2—These tasks make use of the second type of homograph, where pronunciation is the issue. Individuals are asked to find the meaning for each pronunciation of the given words. The pronunciation may depend on which vowel sound is used or differences in syllable stress.

Activity 3—Each item is based on a homophone pair. Individuals are asked to use both members of a pair to make a sentence.

Activity 4—Jokes based on the first type of homograph—words that sound the same and are spelled the same but have different meanings—are presented. Individuals are asked to explain each joke.

Activity 5—Humor items based on homophones are the focus in these tasks. Individuals are asked to explain the use of a homophone and how it created humor in each joke.

Activity Presentation Suggestions

Activity 1 (pages 36–39)

- Encourage individuals to go beyond the meanings that first come to mind by saying things like, "Can you think of another way the word could be used in a sentence?" or "Now try to start (or end) a sentence with the word."

- Discuss the meaning exemplified by each sentence given for a word.

- Encourage individuals to use a dictionary to find additional meanings for a given word.

Activity 2 (pages 40–43)

- Model the pronunciation variations of the word pairs.

- Have individuals think of additional words that change meaning when vowel or syllable stress changes are made.

Activity 3 (pages 44–47)

- Encourage individuals to make original, whimsical sentences using homophone pairs.

- Discuss spelling differences in each pair. Point out how the same sound can be spelled in different ways (e.g., *dough* and *doe, fore* and *four).*

- Have a dictionary available so individuals can look up unfamiliar words before incorporating a homophone pair into a sentence.

- Explain that either member of a homophone pair can be used first in the sentence.

Activities 4 and 5 (pages 48–57 and 58–62)

- Use verbal mediation, brainstorming, and thinking aloud techniques when discussing the questions that follow each item—this will establish a framework for appropriate responses. For a description of each of these techniques, refer to pages 25–26.

- Stress the importance of searching for any context clues that may be available in the jokes. Explain and demonstrate the importance of context clues in interpreting the meaning of a word.

- Have individuals read a joke and then paraphrase what is actually being said. This technique generally helps to clarify the meaning of the joke.

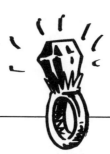

Developing Sentences for Multiple-Meaning Words

Each item in this activity contains a word that has two or more meanings. For example, *ring* can mean "a piece of jewelry worn on a finger," "the sound a bell makes," or "a place where boxers fight." Check out the example below. Then complete the items that follow.

Example

fair

I went to the fair with my sister.

She had a fair complexion.

The weather tomorrow will be fair.

His grade on the test was just fair.

Directions

Write at least two sentences that show different meanings for each word.

1. *fly*

2. *long*

3. *light*

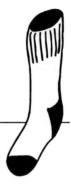

Activity 1

Developing Sentences
for Multiple-Meaning Words

Directions

Write at least two sentences that show different meanings for each word.

1. *slip*

2. *tire*

3. *sock*

4. *kind*

5. *rock*

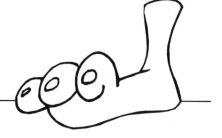

Activity 1

Developing Sentences for Multiple-Meaning Words

Directions

Write at least two sentences that show different meanings for each word.

1. *foot*

2. *break*

3. *class*

4. *grave*

5. *rich*

Activity 1

Developing Sentences for Multiple-Meaning Words

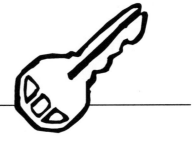

Directions

Write at least two sentences that show different meanings for each word.

1. *key*

2. *like*

3. *track*

4. *run*

5. *back*

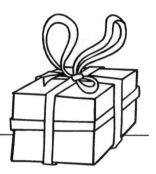

Multiple-Meaning Words with Two Pronunciations

Each item in this activity has a word that can be pronounced in two ways. Each pronunciation has a different meaning. Check out the examples below. Then complete the items that follow.

Examples

*bow—The singer's **bow** fell from her hair when she took a **bow.***
a. bow: *a decorative ribbon placed in the hair, on clothing, and on gift boxes*
b. bow: *to bend the head or upper body forward*

*record—The coach told me to **record** how many times our team broke the **record.***
a. record: *to set down in writing*
b. record: *an attested and certified top performance*

Directions

Provide the meaning for each way the word is pronounced.

1. *present—Sue was selected to **present** the **present** to Tom.*

    a. present:

    b. present:

2. *lead—He tried to **lead** off with a joke, but it fell like a **lead** balloon.*

    a. lead:

    b. lead:

3. *produce—The farm used to **produce produce.***

    a. produce:

    b. produce:

Activity 2

Multiple-Meaning Words with Two Pronunciations

Directions

Homographs in this activity are words that are spelled the same but have two different pronunciations. In each sentence, provide the meaning for each way the word is pronounced.

1. *dove—The **dove dove** into the bushes when it heard the loud noise.*

   a. dove:

   b. dove:

2. *object—I hope you do not **object** to the size and shape of this **object.***

   a. object:

   b. object:

3. *does—The buck **does** funny things when the **does** are present.*

   a. does:

   b. does:

4. *desert—After walking for hours in the hot **desert**, Pierre decided to **desert** the team.*

   a. desert:

   b. desert:

5. *project—The figures he used to **project** the cost of the **project** were incorrect.*

   a. project:

   b. project:

Multiple-Meaning
Words with Two Pronunciations

Directions

Homographs in this activity are words that are spelled the same but have two different pronunciations. In each sentence, provide the meaning for each way the word is pronounced.

1. *wound—He **wound** the bandage around the **wound.***

    a. wound:

    b. wound:

2. *refuse—The garbage dump was so full it had to **refuse** our **refuse.***

    a. refuse:

    b. refuse:

3. *bass—Our **bass** drummer went fishing and caught a large **bass.***

    a. bass:

    b. bass:

4. *row—There was a **row** among the oarsmen about how to **row** the boat.*

    a. row:

    b. row:

5. *close—They were sitting **close** to the door when I asked them to **close** it.*

    a. close:

    b. close:

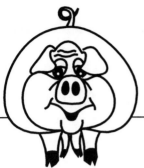

Activity 2

Multiple-Meaning Words with Two Pronunciations

Directions

Homographs in this activity are words that are spelled the same but have two different pronunciations. In each sentence, provide the meaning for each way the word is pronounced.

1. *sow—To help with the planting, the farmer taught his **sow** to **sow** seeds.*

   a. sow:

   b. sow:

2. *wind—The **wind** was too strong to **wind** the sail.*

   a. wind:

   b. wind:

3. *number—After a **number** of injections, his jaw got **number**.*

   a. number:

   b. number:

4. *subject—I had to **subject** the **subject** to a series of tests.*

   a. subject:

   b. subject:

5. *tear—After seeing the **tear** in my new pants, I shed a **tear**.*

   a. tear:

   b. tear:

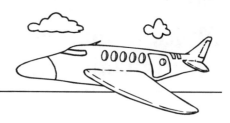

Activity 3: Introductory Activity Page

Using Homophones in Sentences

Another type of multiple-meaning word is a homophone. *Homophones* are words that sound alike but have different meanings and different spellings. For example, *steal* (to take something without asking or paying) and *steel* (an alloy made from iron and carbon) make a homophone word pair. Homophones can be tricky, so it is important to notice the spellings of these types of words. Check out the examples below. Then complete the items that follow.

Examples

flea/flee—The flea saw the bug spray and decided to flee.

bore/boar—We thought the trip to the zoo was a bore until we saw the boar.

Directions

For each homophone word pair, write one sentence that contains both words.

1. *seas/seize*

2. *plain/plane*

3. *made/maid*

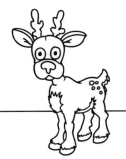

Activity 3

Using Homophones in Sentences

Directions

Homophones are words that sound alike but have different meanings and different spellings. For each homophone word pair, write one sentence that contains both words.

1. _here/hear_

2. _deer/dear_

3. _leek/leak_

4. _reel/real_

5. _weak/week_

6. _foul/fowl_

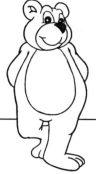

Using Homophones in Sentences

Directions

Homophones are words that sound alike but have different meanings and different spellings. For each homophone word pair, write one sentence that contains both words.

1. *bare/bear*

2. *seem/seam*

3. *write/right*

4. *mail/male*

5. *peek/peak*

6. *vial/vile*

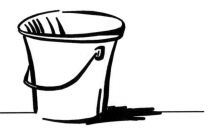

Activity 3

Using Homophones in Sentences

Directions

Homophones are words that sound alike but have different meanings and different spellings. For each homophone word pair, write one sentence that contains both words.

1. _all/awl_

2. _pail/pale_

3. _tier/tear_

4. _seller/cellar_

5. _heel/heal_

6. _need/knead_

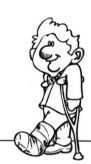

Activity 4: Introductory Activity Page

Multiple-Meaning Words and Humor

A *homograph* is a word that sounds the same and is spelled the same as another word but has a different meaning. For each item, find the word that has more than one meaning and figure out each way it is being used. Look for clues that can help you determine each meaning. The clues can be in any part of the item. Check out the example below. Then complete the items that follow.

Example

Q. Were you ever in a play?   **A.** No, but my foot was in a cast.

   a. Which word in the answer can be used in two ways?   *cast*

   b. What does it mean here?   *a set of actors*

   c. What else can it mean?   *a plaster or plastic mold used to set a broken bone*

   d. Which words or phrases in the question give you a clue to one of the meanings?   *in a play*

Directions

Read each joke and answer the questions that follow.

1. **Man in a restaurant:** I'll have the lamb chops, and please make them lean.
   Waiter: Make them lean? The chef will be lucky if he can get them to stand up.

   a. Which word in this joke can have two meanings?

   b. What does the man mean?

   c. What does the waiter think the man means?

   d. Which words or phrases give you a clue to each meaning?

2. **Q.** Why was Cinderella such a bad basketball player?
   A. She had a pumpkin for a coach.

   a. Which word in the answer can have two meanings?

   b. What does it mean here?

   c. What else can it mean?

   d. Which words or phrases give you a clue to each meaning?

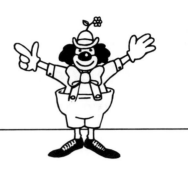

Multiple-Meaning Words and Humor

Directions

In this activity, multiple-meaning words that sound the same and are spelled the same as other words are being used to make jokes. Read each joke and answer the questions that follow.

1. **Q.** Why didn't the monster eat the circus clown?   **A.** Because he tasted funny.

   a. Which word in the answer can have two meanings?

   b. What does it mean here?

   c. What else can it mean?

   d. Which words or phrases give you a clue to each meaning?

2. **Nurse:** Doctor, there is an invisible man in the waiting room.
   Doctor: Tell him I can't see him.

   a. Which word in the doctor's answer can have two meanings?

   b. What does it mean here?

   c. What else can it mean?

   d. Which words or phrases give you a clue to each meaning?

3. **Phil:** Is Frank Walls there?
   Lil: No.
   Phil: Is Pete Walls there?
   Lil: No.
   Phil: Are there any Walls there?
   Lil: No.
   Phil: Then what holds the roof up?

   a. Which word in this joke can have two meanings?

   b. What are the two meanings?

   c. Which words or phrases give you a clue to each meaning?

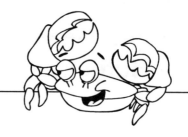

Activity 4

Multiple-Meaning Words and Humor

Directions

In this activity, multiple-meaning words that sound the same and are spelled the same as other words are being used to make jokes. Read each joke and answer the questions that follow.

1. **Q.** Why did Spot go to school?   **A.** He wanted to be teacher's pet.

   a. Which word in the answer can have two meanings?

   b. What does it mean here?

   c. What else can it mean?

   d. Which words or phrases give you a clue to each meaning?

2. **Customer:** Waiter, do you serve crabs here?
   Waiter: Certainly, sir. We serve everybody.

   a. Which word in the customer's question can have two meanings?

   b. What does the customer mean?

   c. What does the waiter think the customer means?

   d. Which words or phrases in the waiter's response give you a clue to his interpretation?

3. **Tina:** Did anyone laugh when you fell on the ice?
   Lena: No, but the ice made some awful cracks.

   a. Which word in Lena's response can have two meanings?

   b. What does it mean here?

   c. What else can it mean?

   d. Which words or phrases give you a clue to each meaning?

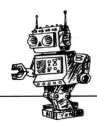

Activity 4

Multiple-Meaning Words and Humor

Directions

In this activity, multiple-meaning words that sound the same and are spelled the same as other words are being used to make jokes. Read each joke and answer the questions that follow.

1. **Stan:** How do you make a horse fast?   **Ollie:** Don't give him anything to eat.

   a. Which word in the question can have two meanings?

   b. What does Stan mean?

   c. What does Ollie think Stan means?

   d. Which words or phrases in Ollie's answer give you a clue to his thinking?

2. **Q.** How do you measure a snake?   **A.** In inches because it has no feet.

   a. Which word in the answer can have two meanings?

   b. What does it mean here?

   c. What else can it mean?

   d. Which words or phrases give you a clue to each meaning?

3. **Q.** What is a robot's favorite snack?   **A.** Computer chips.

   a. Which word in the answer can have two meanings?

   b. What does it mean here?

   c. What else can it mean?

   d. Which words or phrases give you a clue to each meaning?

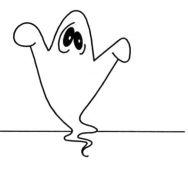

Multiple-Meaning Words and Humor

Directions

In this activity, multiple-meaning words that sound the same and are spelled the same as other words are being used to make jokes. Read each joke and answer the questions that follow.

1. A man was delighted when his son became engaged to a highly regarded lawyer named Jane Price. His friend remarked, "I'm glad to see you got a good Price for your son."

   a. Which word in this joke can have two meanings?

   b. What does it mean here?

   c. What else can it mean?

   d. Which words or phrases give you a clue to the first meaning?

2. **Q.** What happens when ghosts get hurt?   **A.** They get boo-boos.

   a. Which word in the answer can have two meanings?

   b. What does it mean here?

   c. What else can it mean?

   d. Which words or phrases give you a clue to each meaning?

3. **Q.** What did the mayonnaise say to the refrigerator?
   A. Close the door! I'm dressing.

   a. Which word in the answer can have two meanings?

   b. What does it mean here?

   c. What else can it mean?

   d. Which words or phrases give you a clue to each meaning?

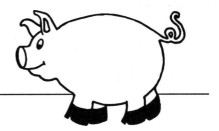

Activity 4

Multiple-Meaning Words and Humor

Directions

In this activity, multiple-meaning words that sound the same and are spelled the same as other words are being used to make jokes. Read each joke and answer the questions that follow.

1. **Larry:** Tom was put in jail for stealing a pig.
   Harry: How did they prove he did it?
   Larry: The pig squealed.

   a. Which word in this joke can have two meanings?

   b. What does it mean here?

   c. What else can it mean?

   d. Which words or phrases give you a clue to each meaning?

2. **Mark:** I'm reading about electricity.
   Mike: I also enjoy reading about current events.

   a. Which word in Mike's comment can have two meanings?

   b. What does Mark mean?

   c. What does Mike mean?

   d. Which words or phrases give you a clue to each meaning?

3. **Q.** Who are the slowest talkers in the world?
   A. Convicts. They can spend 25 years on a single sentence.

   a. Which word in the answer can have two meanings?

   b. What does it mean here?

   c. What else can it mean?

   d. Which words or phrases give you a clue to each meaning?

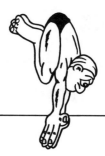

Activity 4

Multiple-Meaning Words and Humor

Directions

In this activity, multiple-meaning words that sound the same and are spelled the same as other words are being used to make jokes. Read each joke and answer the questions that follow.

1. **Q.** What happened to the man who took a dive from a height of 100 feet into a glass of root beer?
   A. Nothing. It was a soft drink.

   a. Which word in the answer can have two meanings?

   b. What does it mean here?

   c. What else can it mean?

   d. Which words or phrases give you a clue to one of the meanings?

2. **Q.** When does Humpty Dumpty play baseball?   **A.** In the fall.

   a. Which word in the answer can have two meanings?

   b. What does it mean here?

   c. What else can it mean?

   d. Which words or phrases give you a clue to each meaning?

3. **Teacher:** Ted, I asked you to draw a horse and wagon. You drew only a horse.
   Ted: I figured the horse would draw the wagon.

   a. Which word in this joke can have two meanings?

   b. What does the teacher mean?

   c. What does Ted mean?

   d. Which words or phrases give you a clue to one of the meanings?

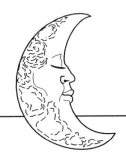

Activity 4

Multiple-Meaning Words and Humor

Directions

In this activity, multiple-meaning words that sound the same and are spelled the same as other words are being used to make jokes. Read each joke and answer the questions that follow.

1. **Q.** Why is reptile music so boring?   **A.** All they ever play are scales.

    a. Which word in the answer can have two meanings?

    b. What does it mean here?

    c. What else can it mean?

    d. Which words or phrases give you a clue to each meaning?

2. **Rudy:** I hear that the moon is going broke.
   Tootie: Where did you hear that?
   Rudy: Well, it said in the paper that the moon was down to its last quarter.

    a. Which word in Rudy's last comment can have two meanings?

    b. What does it mean here?

    c. What else can it mean?

    d. Which words or phrases give you a clue to each meaning?

3. **Q.** Why was the headless horseman always losing his way?
   A. He was absent-minded.

    a. Which word in this joke can have two meanings?

    b. What does it mean here?

    c. What else can it mean?

    d. Which words or phrases give you a clue to each meaning?

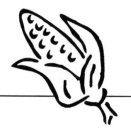

Activity 4

Multiple-Meaning Words and Humor

Directions

In this activity, multiple-meaning words that sound the same and are spelled the same as other words are being used to make jokes. Read each joke and answer the questions that follow.

1. **Joe:** What is the prisoner's name?
   Flo: 5176.
   Joe: Is that his real name?
   Flo: No, that's his pen name.

   a. Which word in Flo's second answer can have two meanings?

   b. What does it mean here?

   c. What else can it mean?

   d. Which word gives you a clue to the first meaning?

2. **Q.** What does a corn doctor cure?   **A.** Earaches.

   a. Which word in the answer can have two meanings?

   b. What does it mean here?

   c. What else can it mean?

   d. Which words or phrases give you a clue to each meaning?

3. **Farm visitor:** What do you do with all the fruit around here?
   Farmer: We eat what we can and what we can't, we can.

   a. Which word in this joke is being used in two ways?

   b. What are the two meanings?

Activity 4

Multiple-Meaning Words and Humor

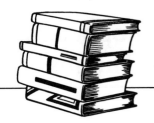

Directions

In this activity, multiple-meaning words that sound the same and are spelled the same as other words are being used to make jokes. Read each joke and answer the questions that follow.

1. **Librarian:** Do you want something light or do you prefer the heavier books?
   Reader: Oh, it doesn't matter. I have my car outside.

   a. Which word in the librarian's question can have two meanings?

   b. What does the librarian mean?

   c. What does the reader think the librarian means?

   d. Which words or phrases give you a clue to the reader's meaning?

2. **Chloe:** People must grow awfully large in England.
   Bess: Why do you say that?
   Chloe: The _London Times_ told about a woman who lost 500 pounds.

   a. Which word in Chloe's last comment can have two meanings?

   b. What does it mean here?

   c. What else can it mean?

   d. Which words or phrases give you a clue to each meaning?

3. **Q.** What do you get if a child stands under a falling piano?
   A. A flat minor.

   a. Which word in the answer can have two meanings?

   b. What does it mean here?

   c. What else can it mean?

   d. Which words or phrases give you a clue to each meaning?

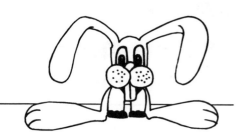

Activity 5: Introductory Activity Page

Homophones and Humor

Homophones are words that sound the same but have different spellings and different meanings. Check out the example below that shows a homophone causing something to be funny. Then complete the item that follows.

Example

Q. Where do chickens go to dance?   **A.** To the fowl ball.

    a. Which word in the answer is used to make this joke funny?   *fowl*

    b. What does the word mean the way it is spelled above?   *a bird of any kind*

    c. How else can it be spelled and what would it mean?   *foul; a ball hit outside the foul lines*

    d. Which words or phrases give you a clue to each meaning?   *chickens, ball*

Directions

Read the following joke and answer the questions that follow.

1. **Q.** Do bunnies use combs?   **A.** No, they use hare brushes.

    a. Which word in the answer is used to make this joke funny?

    b. What does it mean the way it is spelled above?

    c. How else can it be spelled and what would it mean?

    d. Which words or phrases give you a clue to each meaning?

Activity 5

Homophones and Humor

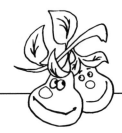

Directions

Read each joke and answer the questions that follow.

1. **Q.** What's a ghost's favorite body of water?   **A.** The Erie Canal.

    a. Which word in the answer is used to make this joke funny?

    b. What does it mean the way it is spelled above?

    c. How else can it be spelled and what would it mean?

    d. Which words or phrases give you a clue to each meaning?

2. **Q.** If twins were a piece of fruit, what kind would they be?   **A.** A pear.

    a. Which word in the answer is used to make this joke funny?

    b. What does it mean the way it is spelled above?

    c. How else can it be spelled and what would it mean?

    d. Which words or phrases give you a clue to each meaning?

3. **Q.** Why was the medieval era called the Dark Ages?
    A. Because it was knight time.

    a. Which word in the answer is used to make this joke funny?

    b. What does it mean the way it is spelled above?

    c. How else can it be spelled and what would it mean?

    d. Which words or phrases give you a clue to the first meaning?

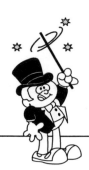

Activity 5

Homophones and Humor

Directions

Read each joke and answer the questions that follow.

1. **Tourist:** The flies are awfully thick around here. Don't you ever shoo them?
   Small-town native: Nope, we just let them go barefoot.

   a. Which word is used to make this joke funny?

   b. What does the tourist mean when he uses the word?

   c. How else can the word be spelled and what would it mean?

   d. Which words or phrases give you a clue to each meaning?

2. **Q.** What happened when the magician did a scary trick?
   A. His hare stood on end.

   a. Which word in the answer is used to make this joke funny?

   b. What does it mean the way it is spelled above?

   c. How else can it be spelled and what would it mean?

   d. Which words or phrases give you a clue to each meaning?

3. Definition of a shopper: Someone who goes buy-buy.

   a. Which word in this definition is used to make this joke funny?

   b. What does it mean the way it is spelled above?

   c. How else can it be spelled and what would it mean?

   d. Which word gives you a clue to the first meaning?

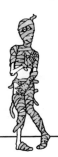

Activity 5

Homophones
and Humor

Directions

Read each joke and answer the questions that follow.

1. **City boy:** Look at that bunch of cows.
   Farm boy: Not bunch, herd.
   City boy: Heard what?
   Farm boy: Herd of cows.
   City boy: Sure, I've heard of cows.
   Farm boy: No, I mean a cow herd.
   City boy: I don't care. I have no secrets from them.

   a. Which words are used to make this joke funny?

   b. What does the farm boy mean when he uses the word?

   c. What does the city boy mean when he uses the word?

   d. Which words or phrases give you a clue to each meaning?

2. **Q.** What do you call a conference of mummies?   **A.** A wrap session.

   a. Which word in the answer is used to make this joke funny?

   b. What does it mean the way it is spelled above?

   c. How else can it be spelled and what would it mean?

   d. Which words or phrases give you a clue to each meaning?

3. **Q.** Why did the cook hurry to the herb garden?   **A.** He didn't have much thyme.

   a. Which word in the answer is used to make this joke funny?

   b. What does it mean the way it is spelled above?

   c. How else can it be spelled and what would it mean?

   d. Which words or phrases give you a clue to each meaning?

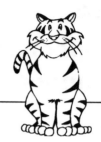

Activity 5

Homophones and Humor

Directions

Read each joke and answer the questions that follow.

1. On a movie marquee: *Revenge of the Tiger*
                          starring Claude Body

   a. Which word is used to make this joke funny?

   b. What does it mean the way it is spelled above?

   c. How else can it be spelled and what would it mean?

   d. Which words or phrases give you a clue to each meaning?

2. **Q.** Why did the sheep keep going straight down the road?
   A. No ewe turns were permitted.

   a. Which word in the answer is used to make this joke funny?

   b. What does it mean the way it is spelled above?

   c. How else can it be spelled and what would it mean?

   d. Which words or phrases give you a clue to each meaning?

3. **Q.** Where can a French monster eat?   **A.** At a beastro.

   a. Which word in the answer is used to make this joke funny?

   b. What does it mean the way it is spelled above?

   c. How else can it be spelled and what would it mean?

   d. Which words or phrases give you a clue to each meaning?

Answer Key

Many responses in this unit will vary. The facilitator must judge the appropriateness of all responses. The answer key is merely meant to suggest some possibilities.

Activity 1:
Developing Sentences for Multiple-Meaning Words

Page 36

1. *fly*

   A bird can fly through the air.

   I'd like to learn how to fly a plane.

   Time seems to fly in the summer.

   Please get the fly swatter.

2. *long*

   I long for the day when I can see you.

   What took you so long?

   There is a long vowel in the word *bay*.

   The dress was too long.

3. *light*

   The paint was a light color.

   Turn on the light.

   I can lift the package; it's light.

   The play was a light comedy.

Page 37

1. *slip*

   She wore a pink slip.

   The boat was still in its slip.

   Joe tried to slip out early.

   He was careful not to slip on the ice.

   The slip of paper was yellow.

2. *tire*

   Lifting the weights seems to tire him.

   Ann realized she had a flat tire.

3. *sock*

   She made a hand puppet out of a sock.

   He said he could sock the ball hard.

4. *kind*

   What kind of bird is that?

   It's a kind of grayish blue.

   She is always so kind to everyone.

   They responded in kind.

5. *rock*

The rock broke the window.

The boat will rock if you stand up.

I like rock 'n' roll music the best.

The girls like to rock at the club.

Page 38

1. *foot*

Rose decided to go on foot.

Bo decided to foot the bill for the party.

There are twelve inches in a foot.

My foot hurts.

2. *break*

Phil tried to break the vase.

Mrs. Lee was given a break on the price.

The role was her big break into show business.

3. *class*

There were 28 students in the class.

He longed to be part of the upper class.

She was so elegant and had a lot of class.

4. *grave*

We placed flowers on the grave.

The doctor had a grave expression on his face.

5. *rich*

The food was too rich for his taste.

King Midas was very rich.

The rug was a rich red color.

Japan is a country rich in tradition.

Page 39

1. *key*

The key opened the door.

Hit the delete key to remove the comma.

The pianist kept hitting the wrong key.

The key for the map was missing.

2. *like*

The sidewalk is like a sheet of glass.

If I like, I can go to the party.

I like lots of cheese on my pizza.

3. *track*

He tried to track down the bear.

Keep track of the time, or we'll be late.

She has a one-track mind.

He walked along the railroad track.

4. *run*

The race was a two mile run.   Sue decided to run for class president.

The sap began to run from the tree.   The car continued to run well after 14 years.

Run these numbers through the computer.

5. *back*

Please scratch my back; it itches.   Mike wants us to back him for team captain.

I'll be right back.   Go to the back of the line.

Find the answer in the back of the book.

Activity 2:
Multiple-Meaning Words with Two Pronunciations

Page 40

1. *present*

    a. to bring to one's attention

    b. a gift

2. *lead*

    a. an introductory comment

    b. a kind of metal

3. *produce*

    a. to bring about; cause to

    b. agricultural products (like fruits and vegetables)

Page 41

1. *dove*

    a. a bird

    b. plunged downward

2. *object*

    a. to feel distaste for something, be opposed to

    b. some material thing that can be perceived by the senses

3. *does*

    a. to behave like

    b. female deer

4. *desert*

    a. arid, barren land

    b. to leave without intent to return

5. *project*

    a. to plan, figure, or estimate for the future

    b. a planned undertaking

Page 42

1. *wound*

    a. to encircle or cover with something pliable

    b. an injury to the body

2. *refuse*

    a. to not accept

    b. trash, garbage

3. *bass*

    a. a low pitched sound

    b. a fish

4. *row*

    a. a noisy disturbance or quarrel

    b. to propel a boat by means of oars

5. *close*

    a. near

    b. to cover or shut

Page 43

1. *sow*

    a. an adult female pig

    b. to plant seeds for growth, especially by scattering

2. *wind*

   a. a natural movement of air

   b. to turn something repeatedly around an object

3. *number*

   a. a quantity of actions, items, or objects

   b. without sensation

4. *subject*

   a. to cause to undergo or endure

   b. an individual whose reactions and responses are studied

5. *tear*

   a. a rip

   b. a secretion of fluid from the eyes when weeping

Activity 3:
Using Homophones in Sentences

Page 44

1. *seas/seize*—You must seize the opportunity to sail the seven seas.

2. *plain/plane*—The inside of the plane was so plain.

3. *made/maid*—Barbara made the maid clean the kitchen again.

Page 45

1. *here/hear*—It's so noisy in here that I can't hear what you're saying.

2. *deer/dear*—Thank you for the picture of the deer, dear.

3. *leek/leak*—The leek soup got watery because it was under the leak in the roof.

4. *reel/real*—Use this reel to catch a real fish.

5. *weak/week*—I became so weak when I didn't eat for a week.

6. *foul/fowl*—The fowl he purchased for dinner had a foul odor.

Page 46

1. *bare/bear*—The bear looked so bare without his hair.

2. *seem/seam*—This seam just doesn't seem right.

3. *write/right*—After getting a gift, the right thing to do is to write a thank-you note.

4. *mail/male*—When I inquired about the Ken doll I ordered, they said the male was in the mail.

5. *peek/peak*—She took a peek at the peak they would be climbing and shook with fear.

6. *vial/vile*—The medicine in the vial had a vile taste.

Page 47

1. *all/awl*—He used an awl to punch holes in all the leather belts.

2. *pail/pale*—That is a pale imitation of a sand pail.

3. *tier/tear*—Lorraine had a tear in her eye when she realized they would be seeing the ballet from the last tier.

4. *seller/cellar*—The coal seller put the coal in the cellar.

5. *heel/heal*—The blister on his heel looked like it would soon heal.

6. *need/knead*—You will need to knead the dough for 10 minutes if you want the bread to taste right.

Activity 4:
Multiple-Meaning Words and Humor

Page 48

1. (a) *lean*   (b) containing little or no fat   (c) tilted to one side   (d) *lamb chops* (which often have fat), *get them to stand up*

2. (a) *coach*   (b) person who instructs players   (c) a large, closed, four-wheeled carriage (d) *Cinderella* (Cinderella's fairy godmother turned a pumpkin into a coach so Cinderella could go to the ball), *basketball player, pumpkin*

Page 49

1. (a) *funny*   (b) different from the ordinary in a suspicious way   (c) amusing   (d) *circus clown, tasted funny*

2. (a) *see*   (b) examine   (c) to be visible to the eye   (d) *nurse, doctor, invisible, waiting room*

3. (a) *Walls*   (b) the sides of a room or building that connect the floors and ceiling or foundation and roof; a person's last name   (c) *Frank, Pete, what holds the roof up*

Page 50

1. (a) *pet*   (b) a student who is treated with unusual kindness and is given special positive attention   (c) a domesticated animal kept for pleasure rather than work   (d) *Spot, school, teacher's*

2. (a) *crabs*   (b) a type of shellfish   (c) ill-tempered people   (d) *we serve everybody*

3. (a) *cracks*   (b) sharp, witty, or sarcastic remarks   (c) narrow breaks   (d) *laugh, fell on the ice*

Page 51

1. (a) *fast*   (b) swift, quickly moving   (c) to abstain from food, not eat   (d) *don't give him anything to eat*

2. (a) *feet*   (b) a unit of length, a measure of 12 inches   (c) the end part of a leg upon which one stands   (d) *measure, snake, inches, because it has no feet*

3. (a) *chips*   (b) part of the hardware of a computer on which information is encoded   (c) small, thin pieces of food   (d) *robot's, snack, computer*

Page 52

1. (a) *Price*   (b) a person's name   (c) value or worth of something   (d) *named Jane*

2. (a) *boo-boos*   (b) a trivial physical injury like a scratch or bruise   (c) sounds ghosts make to frighten people   (d) *ghosts get hurt*

3. (a) *dressing*   (b) putting on clothes   (c) a sauce for a salad or other dish   (d) *mayonnaise, close the door*

Page 53

1. (a) *squealed*   (b) became an informer   (c) to make a shrill, sharp cry or noise   (d) *put in jail for stealing, pig, prove he did it*

2. (a) *current*   (b) a flow of electrical charge   (c) events occurring in the present time   (d) *electricity, events*

3. (a) *sentence*   (b) a grammatical unit of words   (c) judgment that causes a person to be imprisoned for a specified period of time   (d) *slowest talkers, convicts*

Page 54

1. (a) *soft*   (b) moving or falling with little force or impact   (c) soda pop   (d) *root beer*

2. (a) *fall*   (b) a season of the year, autumn   (c) to drop from a high place   (d) *when, Humpty Dumpty*

3. (a) *draw*   (b) to create a likeness or picture   (c) to pull, to move along   (d) *horse and wagon*

Page 55

1. (a) *scales*   (b) a graduated series of musical tones   (c) the external covering of a fish or reptile   (d) *reptile, music, play*

2. (a) *quarter*   (b) a coin worth 25¢   (c) one of the moon's phases   (d) *moon, going broke*

3. (a) *absent-minded*   (b) lost in thought, forgetful   (c) his mind (which was in his head) was gone   (d) *headless, always losing his way*

Page 56

1. (a) *pen*   (b) penitentiary   (c) an author's pseudonym (a fictitious name)   (d) *prisoner's*

2. (a) *earaches*   (b) a pain in ears of corn   (c) an ache or pain in a person's ear   (d) *corn doctor, cure*

3. (a) *can*   (b) to be able to do something; a container in which food is sealed to be preserved

Page 57

1. (a) *light*   (b) of little importance, trivial   (c) having little weight   (d) *I have my car outside*

2. (a) *pounds*   (b) a measurement of weight   (c) English money   (d) *grow awfully large, England, the* London Times

3. (a) *minor*   (b) a person who is not yet an adult   (c) a musical scale   (d) *child, piano*

Activity 5:
Homophones and Humor

Page 58

1. (a) *hare*   (b) a rabbit   (c) hair; covering that grows on one's head   (d) *bunnies, combs, brushes*

Page 59

1. (a) *Erie*   (b) the name of an American waterway   (c) eerie; frightening because of strangeness or gloominess   (d) *ghost's, body of water*

2. (a) *pear*   (b) a fruit   (c) pair; two of a kind   (d) *twins, a piece of fruit*

3. (a) *knight time*   (b) the period of time in history when knights existed   (c) nighttime; the time from dusk to dawn   (d) *medieval era, Dark Ages*

Page 60

1. (a) *shoo*   (b) to scare, drive, or send away   (c) shoe; footwear   (d) *flies are awfully thick around here, let them go barefoot*

2. (a) *hare*   (b) a rabbit   (c) hair; covering that grows on one's head   (d) *magician, scary trick, stood on end*

3. (a) *buy-buy*   (b) to acquire something by paying money; to purchase   (c) bye-bye; a form of goodbye (frequently used by young children)   (d) *shopper*

Page 61

1. (a) *herd/heard* (b) a number of animals of one kind kept together under human control (c) to perceive by the ear (d) *bunch of cows, I have no secrets*

2. (a) *wrap* (b) to enclose with a protective covering (c) rap; to talk freely and frankly (d) *mummies, wrap session*

3. (a) *thyme* (b) a garden herb (c) time; a measurable period during which an action, process, or condition exists or continues (d) *cook, hurry, herb*

Page 62

1. (a) *Claude* (b) a person's name (c) clawed; scraped or scratched at (d) *movie, Revenge of the Tiger, starring*

2. (a) *ewe* (b) a mature female sheep (c) U; a 180 degree turn to go back in the direction from which one came (d) *sheep, straight down the road, turns*

3. (a) *beastro* (b) a small tavern where monsters eat (fictional) (c) bistro; a small bar, tavern, or unpretentious restaurant (a French term) (d) *French monster, eat*

Unit 2:
Multiple-Meaning Phrases

Facilitator Information

Background

Of all the forms of figurative language (i.e., idioms, proverbs, similes, and metaphors), idiomatic expressions are heard most frequently in spontaneous conversation and seen most frequently in written materials. Two-thirds of the English language contains idioms and other ambiguities (Arnold and Hornett, 1990). Unless individuals understand such expressions, they cannot truly understand what is read and heard throughout a typical day. Everyday conversations would sound stilted and unnatural without the use of idioms.

Idioms can be transparent or opaque (referring to the degree to which an idiom's meaning can be figured out from the individual words in the idiom). *Run into a stone wall*, for example, is relatively transparent. The words imply something that is hard to get past and lead to the idiom's meaning. *Break a leg*, on the other hand, is opaque: the meaning cannot be figured out from the individual words. To understand this expression, one must know that *break a leg* means "good luck" in show business.

A *proverb* is an expression that provides a moral lesson, a bit of advice on how to act or think. Like idioms, proverbs can be taken literally or figuratively. Knowledge of proverbs is important because proverbs reflect the beliefs and values of a society. Proverbs expand individuals' knowledge of the society in which they live.

Proverbs, according to the "metasemantic hypothesis," are learned through an active analysis of the words they contain (Nippold, Allen, and Kirsch, 2000). This contrasts with the view that they are learned holistically, as large units, where proverb comprehension reflects the use of rote memory rather than constructive mental activity (Honeck, Voegtle, Dorfmueller, and Hoffman, 1980). While knowing keywords may promote understanding for some proverbs, others may remain obscure until analyzed from other perspectives (e.g., contextual information).

Refer to pages 131–134 in *Saying One Thing, Meaning Another* (Spector, 1997) for a more comprehensive discussion of multiple-meaning phrases.

The Activities in This Unit

The idioms targeted in the Unit 2 activities were selected because they seem to be more commonly occurring in mainstream American culture. The proverbs in this unit were selected from those often found in textbooks, popular media, and spontaneous conversational interactions. Obscure idioms and proverbs were not included within the activities.

Unit 2 contains four types of multiple-meaning phrase activities in the following formats:

Activity 1—Idioms with similar meanings are targeted through a matching task.

Activity 2—Individuals are asked to match proverbs with their definitions. Definitions for all idioms and proverbs in this resource (unless defined in text) can be found in Appendix B. (Given the strong correlation found between word knowledge and proverb understanding [Nippold et al., 2000], a list of keywords is provided for each of the proverb activities.)

Activity 3—Each of the items contains an idiom and its meaning. Individuals are asked to write a paragraph with context clues to illustrate the meaning of each idiom.

Activity 4—Individuals are presented with items in which humor is generated by the manipulation of phrases (mostly idioms). To determine what makes each item funny, individuals are asked several probing questions.

Activity Presentation Suggestions

Activity 1 (pages 79–83)

- Discuss the nature of multiple-meaning phrases with individuals before beginning this unit. Stress the importance of learning the meaning of idioms because they appear in many of the messages individuals hear and read. Mention ideas such as the following, providing examples as needed to illustrate concepts:

    a. An idiom is an expression that can have more than one meaning, depending on the linguistic context (e.g., *give her a hand)*.

    b. Some idioms are easier than others because their meanings can be figured out simply by looking at the words in the phrase (e.g., *my lips are sealed)*.

    c. Some idioms are more difficult to figure out because their meaning cannot be understood from the individual words in the phrase (e.g., *piece of cake)*.

    d. Some idioms have only a figurative meaning (e.g., *falling in love)*.

    e. Some idioms may have several meanings (e.g., *clean up)*

- Enhance learning by providing or eliciting from individuals additional idioms that fit the type of idiom being discussed on an activity page.

- Help individuals visualize idioms (e.g., _hold out an olive branch_ presents an image of offering someone something and this facilitates understanding of the phrase "trying to make peace").

- Reinforce the idea that there is more than one way to say the same thing. Demonstrate that there are several items in the activity that contain as many as three or four idioms with the same meaning.

Activity 2 (pages 84–87)

- Discuss the keywords and their meanings with individuals before presenting each group of proverbs. As an alternative, give the list of words to individuals and have them look them up in a dictionary. Stress the fact that, for many words, there will be more than one meaning.

- Have individuals examine each proverb for context clues. At times, a keyword in the proverb will provide a clue because it is repeated in its definition.

- Ask individuals to determine whether the words that make up each proverb give a sense of its definition.

Activity 3 (pages 88–92)

- Developing a paragraph with appropriate context clues is a rather challenging activity. Thoroughly discuss the examples that precede the activity items. Use the facilitator techniques described on pages 25–27 to assist individuals as they create their paragraphs.

- Have individuals explore the words that compose the idiom. Talk about whether the words might assist in developing clues to include in the paragraph.

- Discuss each paragraph created by individuals. Point out how each clue in a paragraph relates back to some part or all of the idiom's definition.

- Conduct these tasks as a group activity if they are too challenging for individuals to complete on their own.

Activity 4 (pages 93–102)

- Use verbal mediation, brainstorming, and thinking aloud techniques when discussing the examples that precede the activity as well as the questions for each item. This will facilitate the use of cognitive strategies for responding. For a description of each of these techniques, refer to pages 25–26.

- Stress the importance of searching for any context clues that may be available in the humor items. Explain that how an item is interpreted often is dependent on such clues.

- Have individuals paraphrase what is actually being said in an item that is causing difficulty. This can help clarify the meaning of a message.

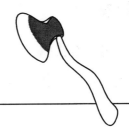

Activity 1: Introductory Activity Page

Idioms with the Same Meaning

An *idiom* is a phrase that does not mean exactly what the words appear to be saying. An idiom's meaning needs to be figured out based on the situation or message. There are times when the same meaning can be expressed by more than one idiom. Check out the examples below. Then complete the items that follow.

Examples

Bury the hatchet means "to try to make peace." What means the same as *bury the hatchet?*

    a. riding for a fall   b. face the music   c. hold out an olive branch

Bawl out means "to scold someone loudly." What means the same as *bawl out?*

    a. read the riot act   b. off the track   c. tell a thing or two

Directions

Read each item and circle the idiom(s) that have the same meaning as the idiom that is defined.

1. *Made of money* means "to be very rich."

    a. snug as a bug in a rug   b. in the money   c. top-drawer

2. *Bend over backwards* means "to do everything possible to please someone."

    a. break your neck   b. go out of your way   c. knock yourself out

3. *Come full circle* means "to return to the original position or idea."

    a. cool one's heels   b. back to square one   c. run around

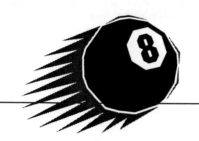

Activity 1

Idioms with
the Same Meaning

Directions

An *idiom* is a phrase that does not mean exactly what the words appear to be saying. Read each item and circle the idiom(s) that have the same meaning as the idiom that is defined.

1. *Blow a fuse* means "to become very angry or upset."

   a. flip your lid   b. lose your temper   c. go ballistic

2. *By the skin of your teeth* means "barely, or by a narrow margin."

   a. hold your own   b. squeak through   c. in great measure

3. *Keep at it* means "to keep doing what you are doing; to keep trying."

   a. hurry up   b. leave no stone unturned   c. plug away

4. *Neither here nor there* means "something that doesn't matter or is off topic."

   a. beside the point   b. come to the point   c. out of bounds

5. *Beat it* means "to go away in a hurry; to leave quickly."

   a. clear out   b. keep the ball rolling   c. head for the hills

6. *Sunday best* means "a person's best clothes."

   a. boiling point   b. glad rags   c. head out

7. *Behind the eight ball* means "in a difficult position; in trouble."

   a. have two strikes against you b. in a hole   c. count off

8. *Chew the fat* means "to engage in small talk; to have a conversation."

   a. pop off   b. play up to someone   c. shoot the breeze

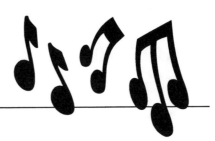

Activity 1

Idioms with the Same Meaning

Directions

An _idiom_ is a phrase that does not mean exactly what the words appear to be saying. Read each item and circle the idiom(s) that have the same meaning as the idiom that is defined.

1. _Call it quits_ means "to decide to stop what you are doing."

    a. throw in the towel   b. knock off   c. on the blink

2. _Face the music_ means "to receive a punishment; to accept the unpleasant results of your actions."

    a. take your medicine   b. pay the piper   c. make your bed and lie in it

3. _Brush off_ means "to be unfriendly to someone; to not talk to or pay attention to someone."

    a. give a cold shoulder   b. lord it over   c. high-hat

4. _Hit the sack_ means "to go to bed and get some sleep."

    a. catch some z's   b. laid-back   c. hit the hay

5. _Fish or cut bait_ means "to go forward with an activity or stop altogether"

    a. first things first   b. head out   c. make up your mind

6. _Worn to a frazzle_ means "to be extremely tired; to be exhausted."

    a. dead on your feet   b. drawn and quartered   c. holdout

7. _Act up_ means "to misbehave."

    a. let down easy   b. raise Cain   c. kick up a fuss

8. _Call it a day_ means "to quit work for the day."

    a. close up shop   b. race against time   c. off the track

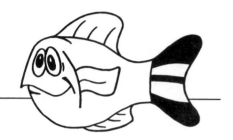

Activity 1

Idioms with the Same Meaning

Directions

An *idiom* is a phrase that does not mean exactly what the words appear to be saying. Read each item and circle the idiom(s) that have the same meaning as the idiom that is defined.

1. *Get ahead* means "to advance or make progress in a certain area."

    a. come up in the world   b. down-to-earth   c. take a hard line

2. *Fish out of water* means "someone who does not fit in or seems uncomfortable."

    a. off center   b. out of your element   c. have a screw loose

3. *It's a cinch* means "something that is very easy; simple."

    a. piece of cake   b. carry the banner   c. draw a blank

4. *Card up your sleeve* means "holding back until just the right time to give yourself an advantage."

    a. bring to a head   b. take to task   c. ace in the hole

5. *High and mighty* means "feeling more important than or superior to someone else; acting proud."

    a. rule the roost   b. stuck-up   c. take down

6. *From scratch* means "to make from the beginning; to start from nothing."

    a. from the ground up   b. live from hand to mouth   c. from hand to hand

7. *Hair stands on end* means "to be very frightened or alarmed."

    a. blood runs cold   b. heart in your mouth   c. run around

8. *At once* means "without delay; immediately."

    a. right away   b. get the jump on   c. get up and go

Activity 1

Idioms with the Same Meaning

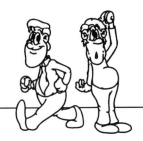

Directions

An *idiom* is a phrase that does not mean exactly what the words appear to be saying. Read each item and circle the idiom(s) that have the same meaning as the idiom that is defined.

1. *Keep under your hat* means "to keep a secret."

   a. don't spill the beans   b. don't let the cat out of the bag   c. mum's the word

2. *Make a long story short* means "to summarize a long story."

   a. talking point   b. keep time   c. in a nutshell

3. *Man in the street* means "the average person."

   a. John Doe   b. John Q. Public   c. man about town

4. *Move heaven and earth* means "to try in every way to get something done; to do everything you possibly can."

   a. hold your own   b. leave no stone unturned   c. pull a fast one

5. *Don't know whether you're coming or going* means "unable to think clearly; confused about what to do."

   a. go whole hog   b. in a bad frame of mind   c. in a fog

6. *Forgive and forget* means "to have no bad feelings about an unpleasant situation; to put an unpleasant event in the past."

   a. let bygones be bygones   b. live and learn   c. put an end to

7. *Leave someone hanging* means "to leave something unsettled or undecided."

   a. up in the air   b. hold the stage   c. on the fence

8. *Make light of something* means "to treat something as if it is not important."

   a. laugh off   b. raise Cain   c. pack off

Matching Proverbs with Their Definitions

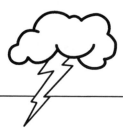

Proverbs are sayings that offer a bit of advice on how to act or think. The words that make up a proverb can, like an idiom, be taken literally or figuratively. For example, the proverb *you can't make an omelet without breaking eggs* can be taken literally to mean "eggs must be broken out of their shells in order to make an omelet." It could also be taken figuratively to mean that "to achieve certain goals one must sometimes incur damage, experience difficulties, or make sacrifices."

Define the keywords listed below. Then complete the items below by matching each proverb to its meaning. The first two have been done to get you started.

Keywords

seen, heard, cross, bridges, before, laid, golden, lightning, strikes, twice

Proverb	Definition
F ____ *All work and no play makes Jack a dull boy*	A. It is extremely unlikely that the same misfortune will occur again in the same set of circumstances or to the same people
D ____ *A little knowledge is a dangerous thing*	B. Don't worry about future events or troubles before they happen
____ *Children should be seen and not heard*	C. Don't spoil something that is good, or something you have, by being greedy
____ *Don't cross your bridges before you come to them*	D. It is better to have no knowledge of something than just a little bit of knowledge, which may cause confusion
____ *Don't kill the goose that laid the golden egg*	E. A command issued by adults to children requesting that they be silent and not interrupt
____ *Lightning never strikes twice in the same place*	F. One should have recreation as well as work to avoid becoming a boring person

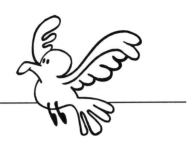

Matching Proverbs
with Their Definitions

Directions

Proverbs are sayings that offer a bit of advice on how to act or think. Define the keywords listed below.
Then complete the items by matching each proverb with the letter that corresponds to its meaning.

Keywords

stitch, time, penny, wise, pound,
foolish, need, indeed, flock, actions, speak, bitten, shy

Proverb	Definition
_____ _A stitch in time saves nine_	A. When you really need help, a true friend will assist you
_____ _Penny wise and pound foolish_	B. It is preferable and more productive to engage in an activity than to just discuss it
_____ _A friend in need is a friend indeed_	C. If you do something when it is needed, you will prevent it from becoming a much bigger task
_____ _Birds of a feather flock together_	D. A person who has suffered from doing something has learned to avoid doing it again
_____ _Actions speak louder than words_	E. People of the same type seem to stay together
_____ _Once bitten, twice shy_	F. Careful in small things but not careful enough in important things

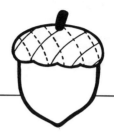

Activity 2

Matching Proverbs with Their Definitions

Directions

Proverbs are sayings that offer a bit of advice on how to act or think. Define the keywords listed below. Then complete the items by matching each proverb with the letter that corresponds to its meaning.

Keywords

curiosity, killed, oaks, acorns, count, before, hatch, early,
catches, silver, lining, half, loaf

Proverb	**Definition**
_____ *Curiosity killed the cat*	A. Don't be too sure that something will happen in the future
_____ *Great oaks from little acorns grow*	B. There is something hopeful in even the worst situation
_____ *Don't count your chickens before they hatch*	C. Part of what we want or need is better than nothing
_____ *The early bird catches the worm*	D. Many great people or things had small and unimportant beginnings, so be patient
_____ *Every cloud has a silver lining*	E. Getting too nosy may lead a person into trouble
_____ *Half a loaf is better than none*	F. A person who arrives early or starts something promptly will gain an advantage of some kind

Activity 2

Matching Proverbs with Their Definitions

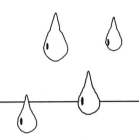

Directions

Proverbs are sayings that offer a bit of advice on how to act or think. Define the keywords listed below. Then complete the items by matching each proverb with the letter that corresponds to its meaning.

Keywords

fits, wear, live, learn, like, look, gift,
pitchers, ears, rains, pours

Proverb	**Definition**
_____ *If the shoe fits, wear it*	A. Don't complain if a gift you received is not perfect
_____ *Live and learn*	B. One good thing or bad thing is often followed by others of the same kind
_____ *Like father, like son*	C. Little children often overhear things they are not supposed to hear
_____ *Don't look a gift horse in the mouth*	D. You learn by experience; the longer you live, the more you will learn
_____ *Little pitchers have big ears*	E. A son is usually like his father in the way he acts
_____ *It never rains, but it pours*	F. If what is said describes you, you must accept it, even if unflattering

Writing Paragraphs That Give Clues

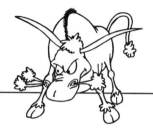

Idioms appear every day in the things you read and the conversations you hear. It's important to practice using idioms so that their meanings become more automatic and make more sense. Check out the example below. Then complete the items that follow.

Example

A bull in a china shop means "a clumsy person who often breaks things without meaning to."

> *Ralph is a very clumsy person. Every time he turns around he bumps into something or he knocks something over. It is dangerous to let him get near anything breakable. He is like a bull in a china shop.*

Directions

Complete the items below by writing a short paragraph containing clues for each idiom that is defined. Be sure to use the idiom in the paragraph you write.

1. *Save your breath* means "to refrain from talking, explaining, or arguing."

2. *Have a sweet tooth* means "to be extremely fond of dessert items or anything made with sugar."

Activity 3

Writing Paragraphs
That Give Clues

Directions

Complete the items below by writing a short paragraph containing clues for each idiom that is defined. Be sure to use the idiom in the paragraph you write.

1. *Rack my brain* means "to try very hard to think of something."

2. *Raise some eyebrows* means "to mildly shock or surprise people."

3. *Tongue-in-cheek* means "to be insincere or joking when making a comment."

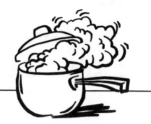

Writing Paragraphs That Give Clues

Directions

Complete the items below by writing a short paragraph containing clues for each idiom that is defined. Be sure to use the idiom in the paragraph you write.

1. *Say the word* means "to give someone a signal to begin."

2. *Have a low boiling point* means "to anger easily."

3. *Her eyes were bigger than her stomach* means "to have a desire for more food than can be eaten."

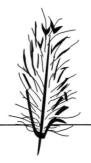

Activity 3

Writing Paragraphs
That Give Clues

Directions

Complete the items below by writing a short paragraph containing clues for each idiom that is defined. Be sure to use the idiom in the paragraph you write.

1. *Feather in his cap* means "an honor or reward."

2. *Fight against time* means "to hurry to meet a deadline or do something quickly."

3. *Clean slate* means "a record of bad deeds or misconduct is forgotten."

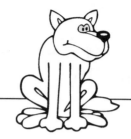

Activity 3

Writing Paragraphs That Give Clues

Directions

Complete the items below by writing a short paragraph containing clues for each idiom that is defined. Be sure to use the idiom in the paragraph you write.

1. *Cry wolf* means "to warn someone of danger that you know is not real."

2. *Have a close shave* means "to barely escape a dangerous or unpleasant situation."

3. *Live and learn* means "to gain knowledge by experiencing life's situations."

Activity 4: Introductory Activity Page

Multiple-Meaning
Phrases and Humor

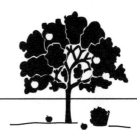

Idioms are used to create humor. Sometimes the meanings of idioms can be figured out by what they are likely to mean in humor items. Check out the example below that shows an idiom being used to make a joke. Then complete the items that follow.

Example

Q. Did you hear what the apple tree said to the farmer?   **A.** "Quit picking on me."

    a. Which phrase in this joke can have two meanings?   _picking on me_
    b. What does it mean here?   _pulling apples off the tree_
    c. What else can it mean?   _criticizing or making fun of someone_
    d. Which words or phrases in the question give you a clue to the first meaning?   _apple tree, farmer_

Directions

Read each joke and answer the questions that follow.

1. **Ann:** Sam the burglar tried to tell the police he was the invisible man.
    Lee: Really?
    Ann: Yes, but the police saw right through him.

    a. Which phrase in Ann's second comment can have two meanings?

    b. What does it mean here?

    c. What else can it mean?

    d. Which words or phrases give you a clue to the second meaning?

2. **Q.** What did the horse say when he finished eating his hay?   **A.** "That's the last straw."

    a. Which phrase in this joke can have two meanings?

    b. What does it mean here?

    c. What else can it mean?

    d. Which words or phrases in the question give you a clue to the first meaning?

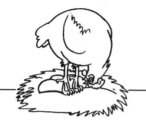

Multiple-Meaning Phrases and Humor

Directions

Read each joke and answer the questions that follow.

1. **Q.** How does a puppet get into show business?
    A. He has someone pull a few strings for him.

    a. Which phrase in the answer can have two meanings?

    b. What does it mean here?

    c. What else can it mean?

    d. Which words or phrases in the question give you clues to one of the meanings?

2. **Rachel:** I heard that you're going to open a bakery.
    Mary Kate: Yes, if I can raise the dough.

    a. Which phrase in Mary Kate's response can have two meanings?

    b. What does it mean here?

    c. What else can it mean?

    d. Which words or phrases give you a clue to the second meaning?

3. **Q.** Why did the hen stop laying eggs?
    A. She was tired of working for chicken feed.

    a. Which phrase in the answer can have two meanings?

    b. What are the two meanings?

    c. Which words or phrases in the question give you a clue to one of the meanings?

4. There was an English aviator who made so many mercy flights that he was knighted by the Queen. Every time he flew over Buckingham Palace he dipped the plane's wings in salute. "Who is that?" asked a visitor. The Queen replied, "That's the fly-by knight."

    a. Which phrase in this joke can have two meanings?

    b. What does it mean here?

    c. How else can the word be spelled and what would it mean?

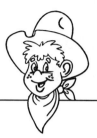

Activity 4

Multiple-Meaning Phrases and Humor

Directions

Read each joke and answer the questions that follow.

1. **Q.** Why did the cowboy aim his gun at the fan?
   A. He wanted to shoot the breeze.

   a. Which phrase in the answer can have two meanings?

   b. What does it mean here?

   c. What else can it mean?

   d. Which words or phrases in the question give you a clue to the first meaning?

2. **Q.** What did E.T.'s mother say to him when he got home?
   A. "Where on earth have you been?"

   a. Which phrase in the answer can have two meanings?

   b. What does it mean here?

   c. What else can it mean?

   d. Which words or phrases in the question give you a clue to each meaning?

3. **Customer:** Why is this doughnut all smashed up?
   Waiter: You said you wanted a cup of coffee and a doughnut and step on it, so I did.

   a. Which phrase in the waiter's response can have two meanings?

   b. What does the customer mean?

   c. What does the waiter think the customer means?

   d. Which words or phrases in the customer's question give you a clue to the waiter's interpretation?

4. **Q.** Why couldn't the orange finish the race?   **A.** Because it ran out of juice.

   a. Which phrase in the answer can have two meanings?

   b. What does it mean here?

   c. What else can it mean?

   d. Which words or phrases in the question give you a clue to each meaning?

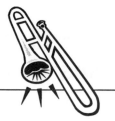

Activity 4

Multiple-Meaning Phrases and Humor

Directions

Read each joke and answer the questions that follow.

1. **Q.** Why are tailors so nervous?   **A.** They are always on pins and needles.

    a. Which phrase in the answer can have two meanings?

    b. What does it mean here?

    c. What else can it mean?

    d. Which words or phrases in the question give you a clue to each meaning?

2. **Q.** What did the sock say to the foot?   **A.** "You're putting me on!"

    a. Which phrase in this joke can have two meanings?

    b. What does it mean here?

    c. What else can it mean?

    d. Which words or phrases in the question give you a clue to the first meaning?

3. **Q.** What is a puppy on a mountain peak?   **A.** Top dog.

    a. Which phrase in the answer can have two meanings?

    b. What does it mean here?

    c. What else can it mean?

    d. Which words or phrases in the question give you a clue to the first meaning?

4. **Q.** How did the trombonist find a place in the marching band?
    A. He horned in.

    a. Which phrase in the answer can have two meanings?

    b. What does it mean here?

    c. What else can it mean?

    d. Which words or phrases in the question give you a clue to one of the meanings?

Multiple-Meaning Phrases and Humor

Directions

Read each joke and answer the questions that follow.

1. **Q.** What happens when the sun comes out at night?   **A.** Oh, that'll be the day.

   a. Which phrase in the answer can have two meanings?

   b. What are the two meanings?

   c. Which words or phrases in the question give you a clue to one of the meanings?

2. **Q.** What happens to a fast witch on a slow broom?   **A.** She flies off the handle.

   a. Which phrase in the answer can have two meanings?

   b. What does it mean here?

   c. What else can it mean?

   d. Which words or phrases in the question give you a clue to the first meaning?

3. **Laura:** What kind of work do you do?
   Ann: I manufacture pencils.
   Laura: How do you like it?
   Ann: It has its good points.

   a. Which phrase in this joke can have two meanings?

   b. What does it mean here?

   c. What else can it mean?

   d. Which words or phrases give you a clue to the second meaning?

4. **Q.** What do you get when you cross a monster with a silent owl?
   A. A thing that scares people and doesn't give a hoot.

   a. Which phrase in the answer can have two meanings?

   b. What does it mean here?

   c. What else can it mean?

   d. Which words or phrases in the question give you a clue to the first meaning?

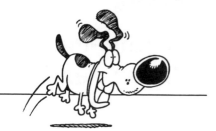

Activity 4

Multiple-Meaning Phrases and Humor

Directions

Read each joke and answer the questions that follow.

1. **Q.** Why do great bowlers play slowly?   **A.** Because they have time to spare.

   a. Which phrase in the answer can have two meanings?

   b. What are the two meanings?

   c. Which words or phrases in the question give you a clue to each meaning?

2. **Q.** Did you hear about the dog that went to a flea circus?   **A.** He stole the show.

   a. Which phrase in the answer can have two meanings?

   b. What are the two meanings?

   c. Which words or phrases give you a clue to each meaning?

3. **Jack:** Oh great! Teacher said we would have a test today, rain or shine.
   Jill: What's so great about that?
   Jack: It's snowing.

   a. Which phrase in Jack's first comment can have two meanings?

   b. What does Jack take it to mean?

   c. What does it really mean?

4. **Q.** What would happen if you cut off your left side?   **A.** You'd be all right.

   a. Which phrase in the answer can have two meanings?

   b. What are the two meanings?

   c. Which words or phrases in the question give you a clue to one of the meanings?

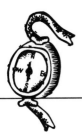

Multiple-Meaning Phrases and Humor

Directions

Read each joke and answer the questions that follow.

1. **Q.** What happened to the farmer who fell down the well?
   A. He kicked the bucket.

   a. Which phrase in this joke can have two meanings?

   b. What are the two meanings?

   c. Which words or phrases in the question give you a clue to one of the meanings?

2. **Q.** Why does Danny always carry around a compass?
   A. So he'll know whether he's coming or going.

   a. Which phrase in the answer can have two meanings?

   b. What does it mean here?

   c. What else can it mean?

   d. Which words or phrases in the question give you a clue to the first meaning?

3. **Q.** What did the mother cabbage say to her son when he told a lie?
   A. "You'd better turn over a new leaf."

   a. Which phrase in the answer can have two meanings?

   b. What does it mean here?

   c. What else can it mean?

   d. Which words or phrases in the question give you a clue to each meaning?

4. **Q.** What is the best way to keep your cool?   **A.** Put ice cubes in your pocket.

   a. Which phrase in the question can have two meanings?

   b. What does it mean here?

   c. What else can it mean?

   d. Which words or phrases in the answer give you a clue for the first meaning?

Activity 4

Multiple-Meaning Phrases and Humor

Directions

Read each joke and answer the questions that follow.

1. Name of a shop that repairs clocks and watches: It's about Time

    a. Which phrase in this joke can have two meanings?

    b. What does it mean here?

    c. What else can it mean?

    d. Which words or phrases give you a clue to the first meaning?

2. **Q.** What did the helmet say to the football player?
   A. "You're putting me on."

    a. Which phrase in this joke can have two meanings?

    b. What does it mean here?

    c. What else can it mean?

    d. Which words or phrases in the question give you a clue to the first meaning?

3. **Angry Buyer:** This car won't go up hills, and you said it was a fine machine.
   Auto Dealer: I said on the level it's a fine machine.

    a. Which phrase in the auto dealer's response can have two meanings?

    b. What does the auto dealer mean?

    c. What does the angry buyer think he means?

    d. Which words or phrases in the buyer's comment give you a clue to each meaning?

4. **Q.** Did you hear about the pelican that switched from herring to sardines?
   A. The larger fish didn't fit the bill.

    a. Which phrase in this joke can have two meanings?

    b. What are the two meanings?

    c. Which words or phrases give you a clue to one of the meanings?

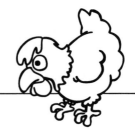

Activity 4

Multiple-Meaning Phrases and Humor

Directions

Read each joke and answer the questions that follow.

1. **Q.** Why was the tow-truck driver arrested when he hitched a racing car to his truck?
   A. They said he was trying to pull a fast one.

   a. Which phrase in the answer can have two meanings?

   b. What are the two meanings?

   c. Which words or phrases in the question give you clues to each meaning?

2. **Q.** Did you hear about the chicken that stopped halfway across the road?
   A. She wanted to lay it on the line.

   a. Which phrase in the answer can have two meanings?

   b. What does it mean here?

   c. What else can it mean?

   d. Which words or phrases in the question give you a clue to the first meaning?

3. **Q.** What will happen if you eat yeast and shoe polish?
   A. You will rise and shine.

   a. Which phrase in the answer can have two meanings?

   b. What does it mean here?

   c. What else can it mean?

   d. Which words or phrases in the question give you a clue to the first meaning?

4. Q. What did George Washington's father say when George brought home his report card?
   A. "Why did you go down in history?"

   a. Which phrase in the answer can have two meanings?

   b. What does it mean here?

   c. What else can it mean?

   d. Which words or phrases in the question give you clues to each meaning?

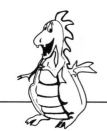

Activity 4

Multiple-Meaning Phrases and Humor

Directions

Read each joke and answer the questions that follow.

1. A group of brave souls were having their first lesson in skydiving. "What if the chute doesn't open?" asked one. "That," said the instructor grimly, "is what we call jumping to a conclusion."

   a. Which phrase in this joke can have two meanings?

   b. What does it mean here?

   c. What else can it mean?

   d. Which words or phrases give you a clue to the first meaning?

2. **Q.** When a dragon is breathing fire, how can you calm him down?
   A. Throw water at him and he will let off steam.

   a. Which phrase in the answer can have two meanings?

   b. What are the two meanings?

   c. Which words or phrases give you a clue to each meaning?

3. **Q.** Why shouldn't you listen to people who just came out of the pool?
   A. Because they are all wet.

   a. Which phrase in the answer can have two meanings?

   b. What are the two meanings?

   c. Which words or phrases in the question give you a clue to each meaning?

4. **Sarah:** Did you hear about the man who fell into the lens-grinding machine?
   Carol: What happened to him?
   Sarah: He made a spectacle of himself.

   a. Which phrase in this joke can have two meanings?

   b. What are the two meanings?

   c. Which words or phrases give you a clue to one of the meanings?

Answer Key

Activity 1:
Idioms with the Same Meaning

Page 79

1. b 2. a, b, c 3. b

Page 80

1. a, b, c 2. b 3. b, c 4. a 5. a, c 6. b 7. a, b 8. c

Page 81

1. a, b 2. a, b, c 3. a 4. a, c 5. c 6. a 7. b, c 8. a

Page 82

1. a 2. b 3. a 4. c 5. b 6. a 7. a, b 8. a

Page 83

1. a, b, c 2. c 3. b 4. b 5. c 6. a, c 7. a, c 8. a

Activity 2:
Matching Proverbs with Their Definitions

Page 84

F, D, E, B, C, A

Page 85

C, F, A, E, B, D

Page 86

E, D, A, F, B, C

Page 87

F, D, E, A, C, B

Activity 3:
Writing Paragraphs That Give Clues

The facilitator should determine the adequacy and appropriateness of the responses for this activity.

Activity 4:
Multiple-Meaning Phrases and Humor

Page 93

1. (a) *saw right through him*   (b) to realize the falseness of something; to understand or detect the true nature of someone or something   (c) he was not visible to the eye   (d) *the invisible man*

2. (a) *that's the last straw*   (b) the final stalk of hay   (c) the last little burden or problem that causes everything to collapse   (d) *horse, finished eating his hay*

Page 94

1. (a) *pull a few strings*   (b) to secretly use influence and power, especially with people in charge or with people who have important jobs, to do or get something; to make use of friends to gain your wishes   (c) to pull the strings that are attached to a puppet (i.e., a marionette)   (d) *puppet*

2. (a) *raise the dough*   (b) to solicit money for a particular project   (c) to add yeast or baking powder to dough to make it rise   (d) *bakery*

3. (a) *working for chicken feed*   (b) working for a very small amount of money; working for the grain that is fed to chickens   (c) *hen*

4. (a) *fly-by knight*   (b) a knight who salutes a queen by dipping his airplane wings whenever he flies over her palace   (c) fly-by-night; irresponsible, unreliable, or untrustworthy; set up to make a lot of money in a hurry and then move along so customers can't find you to complain about your poor work or product

Page 95

1. (a) *shoot the breeze*   (b) to shoot bullets at the fan   (c) to spend some time chatting; to talk   (d) *aim his gun*

2. (a) *where on earth have you been*   (b) what part of the planet Earth   (c) where in fact, really   (d) *E.T.'s mother*

3. (a) *step on it*   (b) to hurry up, go faster   (c) to put the doughnut under his shoe and step on it   (d) *all smashed up*

4. (a) *ran out of juice*   (b) no more energy or strength   (c) ran out of the juice in the orange   (d) *couldn't, orange, finish the race*

Page 96

1. (a) *on pins and needles*   (b) worried and nervous   (c) always have lots of pins and needles around for their work and some may be sat on   (d) *tailors, nervous*

2. (a) *you're putting me on*   (b) the sock is being put onto the foot   (c) to exaggerate; to tease; to act as if something were true   (d) *sock, foot*

3. (a) *top dog*   (b) a young dog that is on the top of a mountain   (c) the head of any business or organization; the most influential or most prestigious person in an establishment   (d) *puppy, mountain peak*

4. (a) *horned in*   (b) to try to participate in something without invitation or welcome   (c) he played his horn   (d) *trombonist*

Page 97

1. (a) *that'll be the day*   (b) the sky will be brightly lit as if it were daytime; the day will never come; that will never happen   (c) *sun comes out at night*

2. (a) *flies off the handle*   (b) she goes faster than the broom, so she flies off of its handle   (c) loses her temper; gets very angry   (d) *fast witch, slow broom*

3. (a) *it has its good points*   (b) it has its positive aspects   (c) good points on pencils   (d) *pencils*

4. (a) *doesn't give a hoot*   (b) doesn't make the sound that an owl usually makes   (c) doesn't care   (d) *owl*

Page 98

1. (a) *time to spare*   (b) over and above the amount of time needed; time to knock down all the pins with two balls in a row   (c) *bowlers play slowly*

2. (a) *stole the show*   (b) took all the fleas away on his fur; gave the best performance   (c) *dog, flea circus*

3. (a) *rain or shine*   (b) only under those particular weather conditions   (c) no matter what the weather, the activity or event will occur

4. (a) *all right*   (b) having no left side of the body; well enough, correct, or suitable   (c) *cut off, left side*

Page 99

1. (a) *kicked the bucket*   (b) died; kicked (or hit) a bucket in the well as he fell   (c) *fell down the well*

2. (a) *know whether he's coming or going*   (b) to know the direction he's coming from or going toward   (c) to be confused about what to do   (d) *compass*

3. (a) *turn over a new leaf*   (b) to start again with the intention of doing better   (c) to turn one of his cabbage leaves over   (d) *mother, cabbage, son, told a lie*

4. (a) *keep your cool*   (b) to keep your body temperature at a comfortable level   (c) to stay calm and undisturbed   (d) *ice cubes in your pocket*

Page 100

1. (a) *It's about Time*   (b) a shop's name that indicates what it sells and repairs   (c) it's long overdue; it's almost too late   (d) *clocks, watches*

2. (a) *you're putting me on*   (b) the football player is putting the helmet on his head   (c) to tease or deceive someone; to play a joke on   (d) *helmet, football player*

3. (a) *on the level*   (b) when you are driving on a level surface, not on hills   (c) honest; dependably open and fair   (d) *won't go up hills, you said it was a fine machine*

4. (a) *didn't fit the bill*   (b) didn't fit into the pelican's bill (beak); wasn't exactly right or not the thing that was needed   (c) *pelican*

Page 101

1. (a) *pull a fast one*   (b) to deceive, trick, gain the advantage over someone unfairly; to tow a car that is fast   (c) *tow-truck driver arrested, racing car*

2. (a) *lay it on the line*   (b) to lay an egg on the line that is in the middle of the road   (c) to say something plainly so that there can be no doubt; to tell truthfully; to speak very firmly and directly about something   (d) *chicken, halfway across the road*

3. (a) *rise and shine*   (b) rise like dough and shine like polished shoes   (c) get out of bed and be lively and energetic   (d) *yeast, shoe polish*

4. (a) *go down in history*   (b) get a lower grade than you did previously   (c) to be remembered or recorded; to be remembered as historically important   (d) *George Washington, brought home his report card*

Page 102

1. (a) *jumping to a conclusion*   (b) jumping to your death   (c) judging or deciding something without having all the facts; to reach unwarranted conclusions   (d) *skydiving, chute doesn't open*

2. (a) *let off steam*   (b) to release excess energy or to get rid of physical energy or strong feelings through activity; vapor that rises from a heated substance   (c) *breathing fire, calm him down*

3. (a) *they are all wet*   (b) they have pool water all over them; they are mistaken, on the wrong track, confused   (c) *shouldn't listen to, just came out of the pool*

4. (a) *made a spectacle of himself*   (b) ground himself up as if he were a lens to be put into spectacles (i.e., glasses); made a public scene or disturbance or attracted unfavorable attention   (c) *lens-grinding machine*

Unit 3:
Multiple-Meaning Sentences

Facilitator Information

Background

When multiple-meaning sentences create humor, individuals must determine what the words in a joke appear to be saying and realize which words can be implied to change the meaning. Newspapers, for example, use the least number of words possible in stating headlines. This often leads to ambiguity. Take, for example, the headline: "Police Help Dog Bite Victim." To interpret this comment correctly, the words that are implied must be made explicit—*police help a victim who has been bitten by a dog.* Otherwise it appears to say that the police are helping the dog bite the victim.

Individuals need to recognize and understand multiple-meaning words and idiomatic expressions that often are embedded in multiple-meaning sentences. For example, note the following newspaper headline: "Red Tape Holds Up New Bridge." To grasp both meanings of this headline, an individual must know that *red tape* means "unnecessary bureaucratic routines" or "tape that is red in color." He or she must also be able to realize that *hold up* can have numerous meanings, including "to support" or "to delay."

The Activity in This Unit

All the items in this unit are of the same type—jokes that are a result of multiple-meaning sentences. In order to interpret and explain what makes the multiple-meaning sentence items in this unit funny, individuals are asked questions designed to do the following:

1. Determine what the words appear to be saying
2. Determine the alternate meanings

Activity Presentation Suggestions

Since many of the multiple-meaning sentence jokes contain multiple-meaning words and multiple-meaning phrases (i.e., idioms), techniques suggested in the "Activity Presentation Suggestions" sections on pages 34–35 and 76–78 would also pertain during this unit's activity. Specifically, the following techniques are recommended:

- Explain that at times, it may be necessary to manipulate and rephrase sentence segments (e.g., restating "Police Help Dog Bite Victim" to read: "Dog-Bite Victim Helped by Police"). Have individuals paraphrase ambiguous sentences to reveal their alternate meanings. Model paraphrasing as needed in order for individuals to learn how to use the technique successfully.

- Stress the importance of searching for any context clues that may be available in the jokes. Explain and demonstrate the importance of context clues in interpreting the meanings of multiple-meaning sentences.

- Have individuals explore the meanings of idioms that are not familiar. Discuss the literal and figurative meanings of the idioms. Talk about the words and phrases within the sentences that contribute to a literal or a figurative interpretation of the idiom.

- Use verbal mediation, brainstorming, and thinking aloud techniques when discussing the questions that follow each item. This will facilitate the use of cognitive strategies for responding. For a description of each of these techniques, refer to pages 25–26.

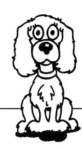

Activity: Introductory Activity Page

Multiple-Meaning Sentences and Humor

Multiple-meaning sentences can have two or more interpretations. To figure out one of the meanings of a multiple-meaning sentence, certain words or ideas must be implied. *Implied* means that the meaning is suggested or hinted at, not actually said. To figure out an implied meaning, you must look at clues that are in the rest of the sentence, rather than just trying to figure out the meaning of each word in the sentence. Sentences that have more than one meaning can be humorous.

Check out the example below that shows a multiple-meaning sentence being used to make a joke. Then complete the items that follow.

Example

Teacher: Joey, what did you write your report on?
Joey: A piece of paper.

    a. What does the teacher's question mean?   *What subject, or topic, did Joey base his report on?*

    b. What does Joey think the teacher means?   *What object, or material, did he write his report on?*

Directions

Read each joke and answer the questions that follow.

1. **Sam:** A dog bit my leg.
   Doctor: Did you put something on it?
   Sam: No, the dog liked it just the way it was.

       a. What does the doctor's question mean?

       b. What does Sam think the doctor means?

2. **Ben:** I lived for a week on a can of sardines.
   Ken: How did you keep from falling off?

       a. What does Ben mean?

       b. What does Ken think Ben means?

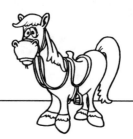

Activity

Multiple-Meaning Sentences and Humor

Directions

Multiple-meaning sentences can create jokes. Read each joke and answer the questions that follow.

1. **Priscilla:** I went riding today.
   Bradley: Horseback?
   Priscilla: Sure. It got back the same time I did.

   a. What does Bradley's question mean?

   b. What does Priscilla think Bradley means?

2. **Boy:** What do you fix shoes with, Mister?
   Shoemaker: Hide.
   Boy: Why?
   Shoemaker: Hide, the cow's outside.
   Boy: I don't care if it is. I'm not afraid of a cow.

   a. What does the shoemaker mean?

   b. What does the boy think the shoemaker means?

3. **Woman:** Can I try on the dress in the window?
   Salesclerk: Well, madam, it's all right with us, but you would have more privacy if you used one of our dressing rooms.

   a. What does the woman's question mean?

   b. What does the salesclerk think the woman means?

4. **Wanda:** My 2-year-old son has a dentist appointment today.
   Wendy: Won't he be afraid?
   Wanda: Of course not. He doesn't know the meaning of the word fear.

   a. What does Wanda mean by her second comment?

   b. What else could her comment mean?

As Far as Words Go © 2002 C.C. Spector
Duplication permitted for educational use only.

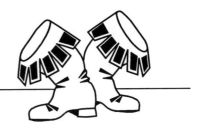

Activity

Multiple-Meaning Sentences and Humor

Directions

Multiple-meaning sentences can create jokes. Read each joke and answer the questions that follow.

1. **Teacher:** Didn't you miss school yesterday, Johnny?
   Johnny: No, not a bit.

   a. What does the teacher's question mean?

   b. What does Johnny think the teacher means?

2. **Pete:** You have your boots on the wrong feet.
   Pat: Well, they're the only feet I have.

   a. What does Pete mean?

   b. What does Pat think Pete means?

3. **Lady:** I would like to buy a pair of alligator shoes.
   Salesman: What size does he take?

   a. What does the lady mean?

   b. What does the salesman think the lady means?

4. **Marsha:** Do you have any wallpaper with flowers in it?
   Clerk: Yes, we do.
   Marsha: Can I put it on myself?
   Clerk: Of course, if you like, but it would look better on a wall.

   a. What does Marsha mean by her second question?

   b. What does the clerk think Marsha means?

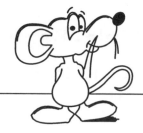

Activity

Multiple-Meaning Sentences and Humor

Directions

Multiple-meaning sentences can create jokes. Read each joke and answer the questions that follow.

1. **Mr. Jackson:** I'm terribly sorry, Mrs. Green, I've just run over your cat. I'd like to replace it.
   Mrs. Green: Well, it's all right with me. But do you think you can catch mice?

   a. What does the Mr. Jackson mean?

   b. What does Mrs. Green think Mr. Jackson means?

2. **Customer:** Waiter, I'm hungry. Please bring me a mashed potato sandwich on rye.
   Waiter: What are you saying? Who would order mashed potatoes on rye bread?
   Customer: You're right. Make it on whole-wheat toast.

   a. What does the waiter's question mean?

   b. What does the customer think the waiter means?

3. **Teacher:** Courtney, spell *mouse*.
   Courtney: M-o-u-s.
   Teacher: But what's at the end of it?
   Courtney: A tail.

   a. What does the teacher's second question mean?

   b. What does Courtney think the teacher means?

4. Sign in a nursery: "All Babies Are Subject to Change without Notice"

   a. Explain the two meanings of this sign.

   b. Which words or phrases give you a clue to the intended meaning of the sign?

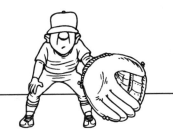

Activity

Multiple-Meaning Sentences and Humor

Directions

Multiple-meaning sentences can create jokes. Read each joke and answer the questions that follow.

1. **Rose:** I feel like a cup of tea.
   Iris: Funny, you don't look like one.
   Rose: I meant, would you join me in a cup of tea?
   Iris: Will there be enough room for both of us?

   a. What does Rose's first comment mean?

   b. What does Iris think Rose's first comment means?

   c. What does Rose's question mean?

   d. What does Iris think Rose's question means?

2. **Tim:** Since I returned from the space flight, I keep seeing spots before my eyes.
   Grace: Have you seen a doctor?
   Tim: No, only spots.

   a. What does Grace's question mean?

   b. What does Tim think Grace means?

3. **Mrs. Brown:** May I have a baseball glove for my son?
   Clerk: Sorry, madam, we don't do swaps at this store.

   a. What does Mrs. Brown's question mean?

   b. What does the salesclerk think Mrs. Brown means?

4. **Doctor:** The best time to bathe is just before retiring.
   Kid: You mean I don't have to take another bath until I'm almost 65-years-old?

   a. What does the doctor mean?

   b. What does the kid think the doctor means?

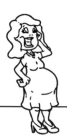

Activity

Multiple-Meaning Sentences and Humor

Directions

Multiple-meaning sentences can create jokes. Read each joke and answer the questions that follow.

1. **Ike:** I hear the men are striking.
   Mike: What for?
   Ike: Shorter hours.
   Mike: Good for them. I always did think 60 minutes was too long for an hour.

   a. What does Ike's response mean?

   b. What does Mike think Ike means?

2. **Betty:** I haven't seen you for a while. Where have you been?
   Bob: I've been away for 30 days.
   Betty: Doing what?
   Bob: 30 days.

   a. What does Betty's last question mean?

   b. What does Bob's last response mean?

3. **Husband:** My wife's in labor!
   Nurse: Calm down. Is this her first baby?
   Husband: No, this is her husband.

   a. What does the nurse's question mean?

   b. What does the husband think the nurse means?

4. **Stephanie:** Did you hear about the turtle on the New Jersey Turnpike?
   Steven: No. What was he doing on the turnpike?
   Stephanie: Oh, about half a mile an hour.

   a. What does Steven's question mean?

   b. What does Stephanie think Steven means?

Answer Key

Activity:
Multiple-Meaning Sentences and Humor

Page 113

1. (a) Did you put some medication or a bandage on your leg?   (b) Did you season your leg to make it tasty?

2. (a) For one week, all he ate was one can of sardines.   (b) He made his home on top of a can of sardines.

Page 114

1. (a) Did you go horseback riding?   (b) Did the horse come back to where they started from?

2. (a) Shoes are fixed with cowhide (i.e., the skin of a cow).   (b) He should go where he can't be seen by the cow.

3. (a) She would like to try on the dress that is being displayed in the store window.   (b) She would like to take off her clothing and try on the dress while in the store window.

4. (a) He's very brave.   (b) He doesn't know how to define the word _fear._

Page 115

1. (a) Weren't you absent yesterday?   (b) Didn't you mind not being in school?

2. (a) You've switched the boots for your right and left feet.   (b) He has the wrong feet (i.e., possibly someone else's).

3. (a) I want to buy shoes made out of alligator skin.   (b) She wants to buy shoes for an alligator.

4. (a) Can I put the wallpaper on the walls by myself?   (b) Can she put the wallpaper on her own body?

Page 116

1. (a) He would like to get the woman another cat.   (b) He would take the cat's place.

2. (a) Mashed potatoes on rye bread is a very unusual kind of sandwich.   (b) The choice of bread to put the mashed potatoes on is wrong.

3. (a) What letter is at the end of the word *mouse*?   (b) What's at the end of a mouse?

4. (a) The babies are changed, one with another; the babies' diapers are changed   (b) *nursery, babies*

Page 117

1. (a) I'd like to drink a cup of tea.   (b) Rose feels like she is a cup of tea.   (c) I'd like both of us to have some tea to drink.   (d) Both Rose and Iris should get into (i.e., sit or stand in) a tea cup.

2. (a) Did you seek medical help?   (b) Have you seen a doctor before your eyes as well as the spots?

3. (a) I'd like to buy a baseball glove for my son.   (b) I'd like to give you my son in exchange for a baseball glove.

4. (a) The kid should bathe just before going to bed.   (b) He should bathe just before retiring from his work or career.

Page 118

1. (a) The men should have to spend fewer hours at work.   (b) There are too many minutes in an hour.

2. (a) What activities have you been doing during the 30 days?   (b) He was in prison for 30 days.

3. (a) Is this the first time your wife is having a baby?   (b) Is this her first baby calling?

4. (a) Why was a turtle on the turnpike?   (b) How fast was the turtle going?

Unit 4:
Sound Changes

Facilitator Information

Background

"Phonological awareness refers to one's explicit awareness of, or sensitivity to, the phonological structure of language. It is the ability to think about, compare, or manipulate the speech sounds in words" (Catts, 1999, p. 17). Although children as young as 8 years of age are capable of grasping some elements of humor based on phoneme level changes, it is not until approximately 11 years of age that they are capable of explaining these changes (Spector, 1997).

Humor items that have a sound added or a sound substituted appear to be easier for individuals to understand than humor items that have a sound deleted. Children and adolescents with language difficulties have significantly poorer comprehension of phonological humor elements than their peers with typical language development (Spector, 1990, 1997).

There is a strong relationship between phonological awareness and reading and spelling skills (Ball, 1997; Clarke-Klein, 1994; Gillon and Dodd, 1995; MacDonald and Cornwall, 1995). Therefore, targeting phonological awareness skills leads to opportunities to strengthen reading and spelling skills.

The Activity in This Unit

The items in this unit were developed to connect phonological awareness with the semantic aspects of language. All the items within this unit are of the same type—jokes that are a result of phoneme changes (referred to as sound changes when directed to individuals). In order to interpret and explain what makes the items in this unit funny, individuals are asked questions designed to do the following:

1. Find the word that has a sound that has been changed

2. Determine how it was changed

3. Determine the relationship of the sound change to the information presented in the joke

All of the humor in Unit 4 is based on making one of the following sound changes in a word:

- taking away a consonant sound
- adding a consonant sound
- changing a consonant sound
- changing a vowel sound

Activity Presentation Suggestions

The following techniques are recommended while using the activity pages in this unit:

- Have individuals focus on how words are pronounced rather than spelled since a single sound can be represented by more than one letter (e.g., /f/ is spelled with an *f* in *fun,* but with a *ph* in *phone* and a *gh* in *laugh).*

- The "funny" word that has the sound change and the real word always sound similar; this fact alone will not be a complete answer to the fourth question in each item (i.e., *Explain why the funny word is used).* Encourage individuals to rely on their world knowledge of the subject to explain the relationship between the words.

- As often as needed, complete items orally with individuals. This will help individuals hear the phoneme changes and facilitate a framework for appropriate responses.

- Stress the importance of searching for any context clues that may be available in the jokes. Explain and demonstrate the importance of context clues in interpreting the meanings of the jokes.

- Use verbal mediation, brainstorming, and thinking aloud techniques when discussing the questions that follow each item. This will facilitate the use of cognitive strategies for responding. For a description of each of these techniques, refer to pages 25–26.

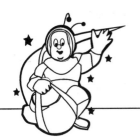

Activity: Introductory Activity Page

Sound Changes and Humor

By making a sound change in a word or phrase, a joke can be created. Sound changes include:

- Taking away a consonant sound
- Adding a consonant sound
- Changing a consonant sound
- Changing a vowel sound

Spelling changes may occur as a result of sound changes. When reading or listening to a joke that is a result of a sound change, focus on how the words sound rather than how they are spelled. Check out the example below. Then complete the items that follow.

Example

Q. Which fairy smelled bad?   **A.** Stinkerbell.

  a. Which word makes this joke funny? *Stinkerbell*

  b. What do you think the real word is? *Tinkerbell*

  c. Which words or phrases give you a clue to why the funny word is used? *fairy, smelled bad*

  d. Explain why the funny word is used. *"Stinkerbell" sounds like "Tinkerbell," who is a fairy in Peter Pan, and "stink" means "to smell bad"*

Directions

Read each joke and answer the questions that follow.

1. **Q.** What do you call a pretty girl using a broom?   **A.** Sweeping Beauty.

  a. Which word makes this joke funny?

  b. What do you think the real word is?

  c. Which words or phrases give you a clue to why the funny word is used?

  d. Explain why the funny word is used.

2. **Q.** When does an astronaut get hungry?   **A.** At launch time.

  a. Which word makes this joke funny?

  b. What do you think the real word is?

  c. Which words or phrases give you a clue to why the funny word is used?

  d. Explain why the funny word is used.

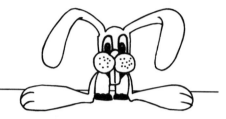

Activity

Sound Changes
and Humor

Directions

By making a sound change in a word or phrase, a joke can be created. Read each joke and answer the questions that follow.

1. **Q.** What do you call a rabbit that is stuck in the mud?   **A.** Unhoppy.

   a. Which word makes this joke funny?

   b. What do you think the real word is?

   c. Which words or phrases give you a clue to why the funny word is used?

   d. Explain why the funny word is used.

2. **Q.** What game is often played in a hen house?   **A.** Chickers.

   a. Which word makes this joke funny?

   b. What do you think the real word is?

   c. Which words or phrases give you a clue to why the funny word is used?

   d. Explain why the funny word is used.

3. **Q.** What's a puppy's favorite soda?   **A.** Pupsi Cola.

   a. Which word makes this joke funny?

   b. What do you think the real word is?

   c. Which words or phrases give you a clue to why the funny word is used?

   d. Explain why the funny word is used.

Sound Changes
and Humor

Directions

By making a sound change in a word or phrase, a joke can be created. Read each joke and answer the questions that follow.

1. **Q.** What happened to the cat that swallowed a ball of yarn?
   A. She had mittens.

   a. Which word makes this joke funny?

   b. What do you think the real word is?

   c. Which words or phrases give you a clue to why the funny word is used?

   d. Explain why the funny word is used.

2. **Mickey:** My cousin is a Russian mouse.
   Minnie: Where does she live?
   Mickey: In Mouse-cow.

   a. Which word makes this joke funny?

   b. What do you think the real word is?

   c. Which words or phrases give you a clue to why the funny word is used?

   d. Explain why the funny word is used.

3. **Q.** What do frogs do after they're married?   **A.** Live hoppily ever after.

   a. Which word makes this joke funny?

   b. What do you think the real word is?

   c. Which words or phrases give you a clue to why the funny word is used?

   d. Explain why the funny word is used.

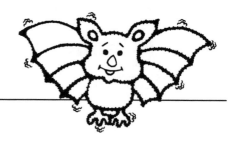

Activity

Sound Changes and Humor

Directions

By making a sound change in a word or phrase, a joke can be created. Read each joke and answer the questions that follow.

1. **Q.** Where does Dracula like to go when he's in New York?
   A. To the Vampire State Building.

   a. Which word makes this joke funny?

   b. What do you think the real word is?

   c. Which words or phrases give you a clue to why the funny word is used?

   d. Explain why the funny word is used.

2. **Q.** Where are you most likely to find bats in your house?
   A. In the batroom.

   a. Which word makes this joke funny?

   b. What do you think the real word is?

   c. Which words or phrases give you a clue to why the funny word is used?

   d. Explain why the funny word is used.

3. **Q.** What is it called when it rains cats?
   A. A downpurr.

   a. Which word makes this joke funny?

   b. What do you think the real word is?

   c. Which words or phrases give you a clue to why the funny word is used?

   d. Explain why the funny word is used.

Sound Changes and Humor

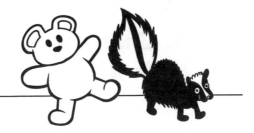

Directions

By making a sound change in a word or phrase, a joke can be created. Read each joke and answer the questions that follow.

1. **Q.** What kind of shoes do mice wear to run away from cats?
   A. Squeakers.

   a. Which word makes this joke funny?

   b. What do you think the real word is?

   c. Which words or phrases give you a clue to why the funny word is used?

   d. Explain why the funny word is used.

2. **Q.** What's a pig's favorite television game show?
   A. Squeal of Fortune.

   a. Which word makes this joke funny?

   b. What do you think the real word is?

   c. Which words or phrases give you a clue to why the funny word is used?

   d. Explain why the funny word is used.

3. **Q.** What do you get when you cross a teddy bear with a skunk?
   A. Winnie the Phew.

   a. Which word makes this joke funny?

   b. What do you think the real word is?

   c. Which words or phrases give you a clue to why the funny word is used?

   d. Explain why the funny word is used.

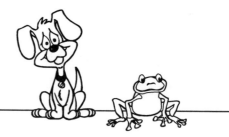

Activity

Sound Changes
and Humor

Directions

By making a sound change in a word or phrase, a joke can be created. Read each joke and answer the questions that follow.

1. **Q.** What do you get when you cross a frog with a dog?
   A. A croaker spaniel.

   a. Which word makes this joke funny?

   b. What do you think the real word is?

   c. Which words or phrases give you a clue to why the funny word is used?

   d. Explain why the funny word is used.

2. There's a scale over there. Go weigh!

   a. Which word makes this joke funny?

   b. What do you think the real word is?

   c. Which words or phrases give you a clue to why the funny word is used?

   d. Explain why the funny word is used.

3. **Q.** What's a duck's favorite party dip?
   A. Quackamole.

   a. Which word makes this joke funny?

   b. What do you think the real word is?

   c. Which words or phrases give you a clue to why the funny word is used?

   d. Explain why the funny word is used.

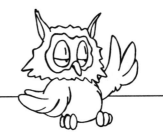

Activity

Sound Changes and Humor

Directions

By making a sound change in a word or phrase, a joke can be created. Read each joke and answer the questions that follow.

1. **Q.** What kind of shoes do reptiles wear?
   A. Snakers.

   a. Which word makes this joke funny?

   b. What do you think the real word is?

   c. Which words or phrases give you a clue to why the funny word is used?

   d. Explain why the funny word is used.

2. Sign at a diet center: "Stop, Look, and Lessen!"

   a. Which word makes this sign funny?

   b. What do you think the real word is?

   c. Which words or phrases give you a clue to why the funny word is used?

   d. Explain why the funny word is used.

3. **Q.** What do you get when you cross an owl with a cat?
   A. An owly cat.

   a. Which word makes this joke funny?

   b. What do you think the real word is?

   c. Which words or phrases give you a clue to why the funny word is used?

   d. Explain why the funny word is used.

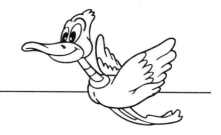

Sound Changes and Humor

Directions

By making a sound change in a word or phrase, a joke can be created. Read each joke and answer the questions that follow.

1. **Q.** What is dog candy called?
   A. Bone-bons.

   a. Which word makes this joke funny?

   b. What do you think the real word is?

   c. Which words or phrases give you a clue to why the funny word is used?

   d. Explain why the funny word is used.

2. **Q.** Is it true that Bill is bald?
   A. No, that's just hairsay.

   a. Which word makes this joke funny?

   b. What do you think the real word is?

   c. Which words or phrases give you a clue to why the funny word is used?

   d. Explain why the funny word is used.

3. **Science teacher:** Today, class, we're going to see a film about waterfowl.
   Bored student: Oh no! Not another duckumentary.

   a. Which word makes this joke funny?

   b. What do you think the real word is?

   c. Which words or phrases give you a clue to why the funny word is used?

   d. Explain why the funny word is used.

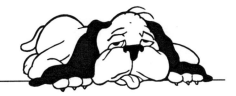

Activity

Sound Changes
and Humor

Directions

By making a sound change in a word or phrase, a joke can be created. Read each joke and answer the questions that follow.

1. **Q.** What is a twip?
    A. What a wabbit takes when it wides on a twain.

    a. Which words make this joke funny?

    b. What do you think the real words are?

    c. Which sound was changed to make the joke?

2. **Q.** What's purple and bites?
    A. A Grape Dane.

    a. Which word makes this joke funny?

    b. What do you think the real word is?

    c. Which words or phrases give you a clue to why the funny word is used?

    d. Explain why the funny word is used.

3. **Q.** What sickness does an old dog get?
    A. Arf-ritis.

    a. Which word makes this joke funny?

    b. What do you think the real word is?

    c. Which words or phrases give you a clue to why the funny word is used?

    d. Explain why the funny word is used.

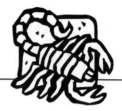

Activity

Sound Changes
and Humor

Directions

By making a sound change in a word or phrase, a joke can be created. Read each joke and answer the questions that follow.

1. **Maria:** Did you hear about the angel who lost his job?
   Tina: No, what happened?
   Maria: He had harp failure.

   a. Which word makes this joke funny?

   b. What do you think the real word is?

   c. Which words or phrases give you a clue to why the funny word is used?

   d. Explain why the funny word is used.

2. **Q.** What kind of bug makes a lot of noise when it's sleeping?
   A. A snore-pion.

   a. Which word makes this joke funny?

   b. What do you think the real word is?

   c. Which words or phrases give you a clue to why the funny word is used?

   d. Explain why the funny word is used.

3. **Q.** What do you call a dog that sleeps all the time?
   A. A schnoozer.

   a. Which word makes this joke funny?

   b. What do you think the real word is?

   c. Which words or phrases give you a clue to why the funny word is used?

   d. Explain why the funny word is used.

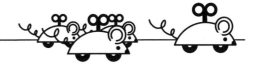

Sound Changes and Humor

Directions

By making a sound change in a word or phrase, a joke can be created. Read each joke and answer the questions that follow.

1. **Q.** How did Mickey help Minnie when she fell into the pool?
   A. He gave her mouse-to-mouse resuscitation.

   a. Which word makes this joke funny?

   b. What do you think the real word is?

   c. Which words or phrases give you a clue to why the funny word is used?

   d. Explain why the funny word is used.

2. Sign on a watch repair shop: "If It Doesn't Tick, Tock to Us!"

   a. Which word on the sign makes this joke funny?

   b. What do you think the real word is?

   c. Which words or phrases give you a clue to why the funny word is used?

   d. Explain why the funny word is used.

3. **Q.** Why do girl mice always beat boy mice in a race?
   A. Because mice guys always finish last.

   a. Which word makes this joke funny?

   b. What do you think the real word is?

   c. Which words or phrases give you a clue to why the funny word is used?

   d. Explain why the funny word is used.

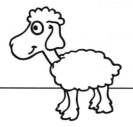

Activity

Sound Changes and Humor

Directions

By making a sound change in a word or phrase, a joke can be created. Read each joke and answer the questions that follow.

1. "Smith," said the coach, "get in there and tackle 'em." Smith went into the game. Soon the opposing team was doubled over with laughter. The game had to be stopped. "What are you doing?" asked the coach. "Why aren't you tackling the other team?" "Oh, tackle!" said Smith. "I thought you said tickle!"

   a. Which word makes this joke funny?

   b. What did the coach really say?

   c. Which words or phrases give you a clue to why the funny word is used?

   d. Explain why the funny word is used.

2. **Q.** What baseball team do ghosts like?
   A. The Toronto Boo-Jays.

   a. Which word makes this joke funny?

   b. What do you think the real word is?

   c. Which words or phrases give you a clue to why the funny word is used?

   d. Explain why the funny word is used.

3. **Q.** If a dog has fleas, what does a sheep have?   **A.** Fleece.

   a. Which words in this joke sound alike?

   b. Which words or phrases give you a clue to why these words are used?

   c. Explain why these words are used.

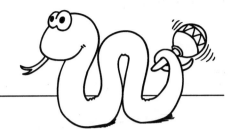

Activity

Sound Changes
and Humor

Directions

By making a sound change in a word or phrase, a joke can be created. Read each joke and answer the questions that follow.

1. **Hal:** I work in a candle company as a trimmer on Saturdays and Sundays.
   Sal: Don't you work there the rest of the week?
   Hal: No. Just on wick-ends.

   a. Which word makes this joke funny?

   b. What do you think the real word is?

   c. Which words or phrases give you a clue to why the funny word is used?

   d. Explain why the funny word is used.

2. **Mia:** Was the baby bird just like his dad?
   Leah: Yes, he was a chirp off the old block.

   a. Which word makes this joke funny?

   b. What do you think the real word is?

   c. Which words or phrases give you a clue to why the funny word is used?

   d. Explain why the funny word is used.

3. **Q.** Why did the rattlers have a reunion?
   A. For old time's snake.

   a. Which word makes this joke funny?

   b. What do you think the real word is?

   c. Which words or phrases give you a clue to why the funny word is used?

   d. Explain why the funny word is used.

Answer Key

Activity:
Sound Changes and Humor

Page 125

1. (a) *Sweeping*   (b) Sleeping   (c) *pretty girl, broom*   (d) Sleeping Beauty is a storybook character who was a pretty girl, and *Sweeping Beauty* sounds like *Sleeping Beauty*

2. (a) *launch*   (b) lunch   (c) *astronaut, get hungry*   (d) astronauts are launched into outer space and *launch* sounds like *lunch,* which we eat when we are hungry

Page 126

1. (a) *unhoppy*   (b) unhappy   (c) *rabbit, stuck in the mud*   (d) a rabbit usually hops and *unhoppy* sounds like *unhappy,* which is what a "stuck" rabbit would be

2. (a) *chickers*   (b) checkers   (c) *game, hen*   (d) a hen is a chicken, and *chickers* sounds like *chicken* and *checkers* combined

3. (a) *Pupsi*   (b) Pepsi   (c) *puppy's, soda*   (d) *Pupsi* includes part of the word *puppy* and sounds like *Pepsi,* which is a brand of soda

Page 127

1. (a) *mittens*   (b) kittens   (c) *cat, ball of yarn*   (d) yarn is used to make *mittens,* which sounds like *kittens*

2. (a) *Mouse-cow*   (b) Moscow   (c) *Mickey, Russian mouse, Minnie*   (d) *Mouse-cow* sounds like *Moscow,* a city in Russia

3. (a) *hoppily*   (b) happily   (c) *frogs, married, ever after*   (d) people who get married are said to live happily ever after and *happily* sounds like *hoppily,* which includes the word *hop,* a frog's way of moving

Page 128

1. (a) *Vampire*   (b) Empire   (c) *Dracula, New York*   (d) Dracula is a vampire, which sounds like *empire,* and the Empire State Building is in New York

2. (a) *batroom*   (b) bathroom   (c) *bats, in your house*   (d) *batroom* sounds like *bathroom,* which is part of a house

3. (a) *downpurr*   (b) downpour   (c) *rains cats*   (d) cats purr and *downpurr* sounds like *downpour,* which is a heavy rain

Page 129

1. (a) *squeakers*   (b) sneakers   (c) *shoes, mice*   (d) mice squeak and *squeakers* sounds like *sneakers,* which are a type of shoe

2. (a) *Squeal*   (b) Wheel   (c) *pig's, television game show*   (d) pigs squeal, *squeal* sounds like *wheel,* and *Wheel of Fortune* is a popular television game show

3. (a) *Phew*   (b) Pooh   (c) *teddy bear, skunk*   (d) Winnie the Pooh is a teddy bear and skunks make a terrible odor when frightened that makes us say *phew,* which sounds like *Pooh*

Page 130

1. (a) *croaker*   (b) cocker   (c) *frog, dog*   (d) frogs make a croaking sound, and *croaker spaniel* sounds like *cocker spaniel,* which is a breed of dog

2. (a) *weigh*   (b) away   (c) *scale, go*   (d) scales are used to weigh someone or something, and *go away* is a familiar phrase that sounds like *go weigh*

3. (a) *quackamole*   (b) guacamole   (c) *duck's, party dip*   (d) ducks quack and *quackamole* sounds like *guacamole,* which is a party dip

Page 131

1. (a) *snakers*   (b) sneakers   (c) *shoes, reptiles wear*   (d) sneakers are a kind of shoe and snakes are a kind of reptile; *sneakers* sounds like *snakers*

2. (a) *Lessen*   (b) Listen   (c) *diet center*   (d) *Stop, look, and listen* is a familiar phrase, and *lessen,* which is what diet centers help you do, sounds like *listen*

3. (a) *owly* (b) alley (c) *owl, cat* (d) *owly*, which includes the word *owl*, sounds like *alley*, which is a type of cat

Page 132

1. (a) *bone-bons* (b) bonbons (c) *dog candy* (d) dogs like bones and *bone-bons* sounds like *bonbons*, which is a kind of candy

2. (a) *hairsay* (b) hearsay (c) *is it true, bald* (d) a bald man lacks hair, and *hairsay*, which includes the word *hair*, sounds like *hearsay*, which is just a rumor

3. (a) *duckumentary* (b) documentary (c) *film about waterfowl* (d) a duck is a waterfowl, and a film can be a *documentary*, which sounds like *duckumentary*

Page 133

1. (a) *twip, wabbit, wides, twain* (b) trip, rabbit, rides, train (c) *w* was used for *r*

2. (a) *Grape* (b) Great (c) *purple, bites* (d) *grape* sounds like *great* and a Great Dane is a breed of dog

3. (a) *arf-ritis* (b) arthritis (c) *sickness, old dog* (d) arthritis is an inflammation of the joints usually affecting older people (and animals), and *arthritis* sounds like *arf-ritis*, which includes the sound a dog makes

Page 134

1. (a) *harp* (b) heart (c) *angel, failure* (d) angels are frequently shown playing harps, and *harp failure*, which sounds like *heart failure*, could be considered a reason for an angel to lose a job

2. (a) *snore-pion* (b) scorpion (c) *bug, makes a lot of noise when it's sleeping* (d) a scorpion is a kind of bug, snoring is a noise sometimes made when someone is asleep, and *snore-pion* sounds like *scorpion*

3. (a) *schnoozer* (b) schnauzer (c) *dog that sleeps all the time* (d) *schnoozer* sounds like the word *snooze*, which means to nap, and *schnoozer* also sounds like *schnauzer*, which is a type of dog

Page 135

1. (a) *mouse-to-mouse*   (b) mouth-to-mouth   (c) *Mickey, Minnie, fell into the pool, resuscitation* (d) mouth-to-mouth resuscitation is given when someone is in danger of losing his or her life, Mickey and Minnie are mice in Disney cartoons, and *mouse-to-mouse* sounds like *mouth-to-mouth*

2. (a) *Tock*   (b) talk   (c) *watch repair shop*   (d) watches in good condition make a tick-tock sound, you talk to someone in a repair shop if your watch is not working, and *tock* sounds like *talk*

3. (a) *mice*   (b) nice   (c) *boy mice, always finish last*   (d) a boy can be called a guy and *mice guys always finish last* sounds like the familiar expression *nice guys always finish last*

Page 136

1. (a) *tickle*   (b) tackle   (c) *doubled over with laughter*   (d) *tickle* sounds like *tackle*, which could lead to someone mishearing

2. (a) *Boo-Jays*   (b) Blue Jays   (c) *baseball team, ghosts*   (d) Blue Jays is the name of a baseball team and ghosts say *boo*, which sounds like *blue*

3. (a) *fleas* and *fleece*   (b) *dog, sheep*   (c) dogs often have fleas, which sounds like *fleece*—the wool covering on a sheep's body

Page 137

1. (a) *wick*   (b) week   (c) *candle, Saturdays and Sundays*   (d) a candle has a *wick*, which sounds like *week*, and Saturday and Sunday are weekend days

2. (a) *chirp*   (b) chip   (c) *baby bird, like his dad*   (d) a bird chirps and *chirp off the old block* sounds like the familiar expression *chip off the old block*, which means someone who resembles his or her parent(s)

3. (a) *snake*   (b) sake   (c) *rattlers, reunion*   (d) rattlers are snakes, a reunion is when people get together after not seeing each other for a long time, and *for old time's snake* sounds like the familiar expression *for old time's sake*

Unit 5:
Switching Sounds
or Words

Facilitator Information

Background

Transposing sounds or words often occurs unexpectedly when we speak. These utterances are called *spoonerisms* and can be amusing. An example of a sound switch is, *I was late because I couldn't find a sparking pot* (parking spot). These transpositions occur because the articulators "jump the gun" and produce a sound that will occur later in the sequence of sounds in a word or phrase, instead of the earlier occurring sound. Sound or word switches can also be intentional, in order to create humor. For example:

> *Q. What's the difference between a hungry man and a greedy man?*

> *A. One longs to eat and the other eats too long.*

Some items that have word switches are based on idiomatic expressions. For example, the idiom *sticking your nose into someone else's business* is the basis for the following item:

> *Nasal spray salesman: A guy who goes around sticking his business into other people's noses*

The Activities in This Unit

The activities in this unit are based on either sound switches or word switches that create humor. To determine what makes "switched" items funny, individuals are asked questions designed to have them do the following:

1. Look for the switch

2. Determine which sounds or words are being manipulated

3. Select and describe the switched items

4. Determine why the switch is made

The activity format throughout this unit is the same, but the humor items have been grouped into Activity 1 (sound switches) and Activity 2 (word switches) to separate the two different types of humor items.

When individuals are asked to explain why sound or word switches are made, a variety of responses could be acceptable. The explanations for why the switches are made should center around the meanings of both phrases presented in the answers of these jokes. For example, an individual should explain the meaning of "trained to run" (e.g., to describe what you do with a race horse) and "runs a train" (e.g., to describe what an engineer does) for the joke:

Q. What is the difference between a race horse and an engineer?

A. One is trained to run, and the other runs a train.

Activity Presentation Suggestions

Activity 1 (pages 147–148)

- Have items read aloud so that individuals can hear the sound switches. As needed, explain the nature of sound switches.

- Have individuals focus on how words are pronounced rather than spelled since a single sound can be represented by more than one letter (e.g., /f/ is spelled with an *f* in *fun*, but with a *ph* in *phone* and a *gh* in *laugh*).

- Stress the importance of searching for any context clues that may be available in the jokes. Explain and demonstrate the importance of context clues in interpreting the meanings of the jokes.

- Use verbal mediation, brainstorming, and thinking aloud techniques when discussing the questions that follow each item. This will facilitate the use of cognitive strategies for responding. For a description of each of these techniques, refer to pages 25–26.

Activity 2 (pages 149–152)

- Alert individuals to spelling changes that may occur as a result of switching words to create a joke (e.g., *tale/tail*). When homophone word pairs are present, talk about how these multiple-meaning words play a role in creating the humor in an item.

- Stress the importance of searching for any context clues that may be available in the jokes. Explain and demonstrate the importance of context clues in interpreting the meanings of the jokes.

- Have individuals explore the meanings of idioms that are not familiar. Discuss the literal and figurative meanings of the idioms. Talk about the words and phrases within the sentences that contribute to a literal or a figurative interpretation of the idiom.

- Use verbal mediation, brainstorming, and thinking aloud techniques when discussing the questions that follow each item. This will facilitate the use of cognitive strategies for responding. For a description of each of these techniques, refer to pages 25–26.

Activity 1: Introductory Activity Page

Switching Sounds to Create Humor

Switching sounds between words can create humor. Sometimes these switches are accidental and something that is said becomes funny. These switches can also be made on purpose to create a joke. Check out the example below. Then complete the items that follow.

Example

Q. What's the difference between a greedy person and an electric toaster?
A. One takes the most, the other makes the toast.

    a. Which words in the answer have switched sounds?   *takes/most and makes/toast*

    b. Which sounds are switched?   *t and m*

    c. Why is the switch made in this way?   *to describe a greedy person and a toaster*

Directions

Read each joke and answer the questions that follow.

1. **Q.** What's the difference between a whale hunter and a happy dog?
   A. One tags his whale and the other wags his tail.

    a. Which words in the answer have switched sounds?

    b. Which sounds are switched?

    c. Why are the sounds switched in this way?

2. Usher in a darkened movie theater: "Let me sew you to your sheet."

    a. Which sounds in this joke are switched?

    b. What does the usher mean to say?

    c. Which words or phrases give you a clue to what the usher means?

    d. Why are the sounds switched in this way?

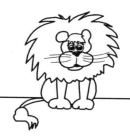

Activity 1

Switching Sounds to Create Humor

Directions

Switching sounds between words can create humor. Read each joke and answer the questions that follow.

1. **Q.** What's the difference between a lazy schoolboy and a fisherman?
   A. A fisherman baits his hooks, and a lazy schoolboy hates his books.

   a. Which words in the answer have switched sounds?

   b. Which sounds are switched?

   c. Why are the sounds switched in this way?

2. **Q.** What's the difference between a lion with a toothache and a rainy day?
   A. One roars with pain and the other pours with rain.

   a. Which words in the answer have switched sounds?

   b. Which sounds are switched?

   c. Why are the sounds switched in this way?

3. **Q.** What's the difference between the place you tie up your horse and a party-giving ball player?
   A. One's a hitching post and the other is a pitching host.

   a. Which words in the answer have switched sounds?

   b. Which sounds are switched?

   c. Why are the sounds switched in this way?

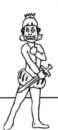

Activity 2: Introductory Activity Page

Switching Words to Create Humor

Switching words around in a sentence can create humor. Sometimes word switches are accidental and something that is said becomes funny. These switches can also be made on purpose to create a joke. Check out the example below. Then complete the items that follow.

Example

Q. What's the difference between a race horse and an engineer?
A. One is trained to run, and the other runs a train.

    a. Which phrases in the answer have words that are switched?   *trained to run, runs a train*

    b. What does each phrase mean?   *taught to move quickly; operates a locomotive engine*

    c. Why is the switch made in this way?   *to describe what you do with a race horse; to describe what an engineer does*

Directions

Read each joke and answer the questions that follow.

1. **Q.** What's the difference between a hungry man and a greedy man?
   A. One longs to eat and the other eats too long.

    a. Which phrases in the answer have words that are switched?

    b. What does each phrase mean?

    c. Why is the switch made in this way?

2. **Q.** What's the difference between a basketball and Prince Charles?
   A. One is thrown in the air, and the other is heir to the throne.

    a. Which phrases in the answer have words that are switched?

    b. What does each word mean?

    c. Why is the switch made in this way?

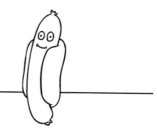

Activity 2

Switching Words
to Create Humor

Directions

Switching words around in a sentence can create humor. Read each joke and answer the questions that follow.

1. **Q.** What's the difference between a watchmaker and a jailer?
   A. One sells watches and the other watches cells.

   a. Which phrases in the answer have words that are switched?

   b. What does each phrase mean?

   c. Why is the switch made in this way?

2. **Q.** What's the difference between a book of fiction and the red light at the rear of a car?
   A. One is a light tale and the other is a taillight.

   a. Which words in the answer are switched?

   b. What are the two meanings of these words?

   c. Why is the switch made in this way?

3. **Q.** Why is a hot dog the best dog of all?
   A. Because it feeds the hand that bites it.

   a. Which two words in the answer are switched?

   b. What expression is the answer based on?

   c. What does the expression mean?

   d. Why are the words switched in this way?

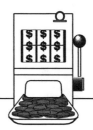

Activity 2

Switching Words to Create Humor

Directions

Switching words around in a sentence can create humor. Read each joke and answer the questions that follow.

1. **Q.** How is an actor in a hit show like a hockey player?
   A. One sticks with the play, and the other plays with a stick.

   a. Which phrases in the answer have words that are switched?

   b. Which words are changed in this joke?

   c. Why are the words switched in this way?

2. At an army post, they put some "one-armed bandits" into the officers' bunkhouses. The slot machines were in the officers' quarters, and soon the officers' quarters were in the slot machines.

   a. Which word in this joke is being used in two ways?

   b. What are the two meanings?

   c. What's another way of saying slot machines?

3. Nasal spray salesman: a guy who goes around sticking his business into other people's noses

   a. Which two words in this definition are switched?

   b. What expression is this joke based on?

   c. Why is the switch made in this way?

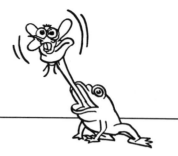

Activity 2

Switching Words to Create Humor

Directions

Switching words around in a sentence can create humor. Read each joke and answer the questions that follow.

1. One of King Arthur's knights charged into an inn. A fierce storm raged outside. "Can you lend me a horse?" he asked the innkeeper. "My steed is too weary to go another step." "Sir Knight," the innkeeper replied, "I have no horse. The only animal I have is that big, old dog in the corner." "Very well," said the knight, "I shall ride him." "Oh no, sire!" the innkeeper cried. "I wouldn't send a knight out on a dog like this."

   a. Which words in the innkeeper's last comment are switched?

   b. Which of these words can be spelled differently to change its meaning?

   c. How else can this word be spelled?

   d. What familiar expression is this joke based on?

2. One frog to another: "Time sure is fun when you're having flies!"

   a. Which words in this comment are switched?

   b. Why are the words switched in this way?

   c. What expression is this joke based on?

3. **Q.** What's the difference between a cat and a comma?
   A. A cat has claws at the end of its paws, and a comma is a pause at the end of a clause.

   a. Which phrases in the answer have words that are switched?

   b. What does each phrase mean?

Answer Key

Activity 1:
Switching Sounds to Create Humor

Page 147

1. (a) _tags/whale_ and _wags/tail_   (b) _t_ and _w_   (c) whale hunters mark their catch with a tag, and when a dog is happy, he wags his tail

2. (a) _s_ and _sh_   (b) "Let me show you to your seat"   (c) _usher, movie theater_   (d) this may have been a "slip of the tongue" or a "spoonerism," where someone switches sounds by accident; this happens to all of us at times, and the result is often funny

Page 148

1. (a) _baits/hooks_ and _hates/books_   (b) _b_ and _h_   (c) to describe a lazy schoolboy and a fisherman

2. (a) _roars/pain_ and _pours/rain_ (b) _r_ and _p_ (c) _roars with pain_—describes what a lion with a toothache does; _pours with rain_—describes a rainy day

3. (a) _hitching/post_ and _pitching/host_   (b) _h_ and _p_   (c) because you tie a horse to a hitching post, and a ballplayer who pitches can host a party

Activity 2:
Switching Words to Create Humor

Page 149

1. (a) _longs to eat_ and _eats too long_   (b) _longs to eat_—doesn't have food or is not allowed to eat; _eats too long_—keeps eating longer than necessary to satisfy a normal appetite   (c) to describe a hungry man and a greedy man

2. (a) _thrown in the air_ and _heir to the throne_   (b) _thrown_—tossed in the air; _throne_—seat for royalty; _air_—substance we breathe; _heir_—one in line to inherit a title   (c) to describe how a basketball can be used and to describe Prince Charles, heir to the British throne

Page 150

1. (a) *sells watches* and *watches cells*   (b) *sells watches*—offers timepieces for sale; *watches cells*—looks at or observes prison rooms   (c) to describe what a watchmaker and a jailer do

2. (a) *light tale* and *taillight*   (b) *light tale*—a story of trivial importance; *taillight*—a light at the rear end of a vehicle   (c) to describe a book of fiction and the red light at the end of a car

3. (a) *feeds* and *bites*   (b) don't bite the hand that feeds you   (c) don't do harm to someone who does good things for you   (d) to describe the kind of dog that nourishes you

Page 151

1. (a) *sticks with a play* and *plays with a stick*   (b) the s was removed from *sticks* to make *stick*, and an *s* was added to *play* to make *plays*   (c) to describe an actor who stays with a dramatic production and what a hockey player uses to engage in a hockey game

2. (a) *quarters*   (b) living space, accommodations; coins, money   (c) one-armed bandits

3. (a) *business* and *noses*   (b) sticking his nose into other people's business   (c) the salesman is selling nasal spray, which one puts into one's nose

Page 152

1. (a) *knight* and *dog*   (b) *knight*   (c) night   (d) I wouldn't send a dog out there on a night like this

2. (a) *fun* and *flies*   (b) frogs enjoy spending their time eating flies (insects)   (c) time sure flies (i.e., goes by quickly) when you're having fun

3. (a) *claws at the end of its paws* and *pause at the end of a clause*   (b) *claws at the end of its paws*—an animal's nails on its feet (paws); *pause at the end of a clause*—part of a sentence where you stop for a moment

Unit 6:
Stress and Pausing Changes

Facilitator Information
Background

Two important elements of a spoken message are stress and juncture. *Stress* refers to the amount of force used in the production of one syllable as compared with another (Nicolosi, Harryman, and Kresheck, 1996). *Juncture* is the way in which syllables or words are joined together in connected speech (Nicolosi et al., 1996). Juncture incorporates stress and pausing elements. Stress and juncture changes can greatly affect the meaning of spoken messages.

Understanding the items in this unit can be difficult for individuals because it requires the coordination of several metalinguistic skills. Word boundaries must be determined, the syllables of a word or a series of words have to be segmented and regrouped, and, at times, sound changes may be needed. All this must be done without the support of underlying meaning (Spector, 1990).

The Activity in This Unit

The activity in this unit contains jokes that are a result of changes in stress and juncture. Since aspects of stress and juncture are nearly impossible to separate from each other, items within this unit are not grouped based on stress changes versus juncture changes. To determine what makes these items funny, individuals are asked questions designed to have them do the following:

1. Select the word(s) the humor is based on

2. Resegment the word(s) to give them other meanings

3. Determine the word(s) that give the best clues to one or both meanings

The word *pausing* is used when referring to juncture on the activity pages throughout this unit. This terminology was selected because it is more familiar to individuals.

Activity Presentation Suggestions

The following techniques are recommended while using the activity pages in this unit:

- Conduct all tasks aloud when first beginning with the activity pages in the unit. Verbalizing the stress and juncture differences in the jokes can lead to increased understanding of the humor.

- Consider exaggerating the stress and juncture patterns until the individual grasps the nature of these items.

- Use the thinking aloud technique described on page 26.

- For some items, it is necessary to redefine the words in a joke by combining rather than segmenting them. For example:

    Q. What would you do if you were starving on a desert island?
    A. Eat the sand which is there.

    Changing *sand which is* to *sandwiches* requires eliminating two word boundaries and resequencing the entire string of words to create a new meaning.

- Point out semantic clues that may help individuals interpret the stress and juncture changes within a joke. For example, highlight the words *starving, desert,* and *eat* in the above joke.

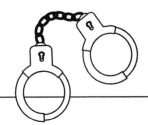

Activity: Introductory Activity Page

Stress and Pausing Changes and Humor

When we speak, we use stress and pausing patterns. _Stress_ is the emphasis you place on a syllable in a word as compared with other syllables. _Pausing_ is the way you separate syllables or words from each other. The meaning of a sentence can change if you change your stress and pausing. Sometimes these changes can make a sentence funny.

The items in this unit are jokes that result from stress and pausing changes. For some items, spelling changes also occur. Check out the example below. Then complete the items that follow.

Example

Q. Did you ever see the Catskill Mountains?
A. No, but I've seen what cats do to mice.

a. Which words can be formed by separating the syllables of a word in the question?
cats kill

b. Which words or phrases in the answer give you a clue to the new words? _cats, mice_

Directions

Read each joke and answer the questions that follow.

1. Bestseller: _Will He or Won't He?_
       by Mae B. Sew

   a. What funny meaning can the author's name have?

   b. Which words or phrases give you a clue to the funny meaning?

2. **Q.** Why are handcuffs like souvenirs?   **A.** They are made for two wrists.

   a. Which two words in the answer can be combined to form a new word?

   b. What is the new word?

   c. Which words or phrases in the question give you a clue to the new word?

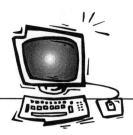

Activity

Stress and Pausing
Changes and Humor

Directions

The meaning of a sentence can change if you change your stress and pausing. Sometimes these changes can make a sentence funny. Read each joke and answer the questions that follow.

1. **Q.** What did the computer say when the spaceship landed on Mars instead of Venus?
   A. "I didn't planet that way."

   a. Which word in the answer can be changed by separating the syllables?

   b. What does the word become?

   c. What is the meaning of the new words?

   d. Which words or phrases in the question give you a clue to why the original word is used?

2. Bestseller: *Reptiles around the World*
                by Sally Mander

   a. What funny meaning can the author's name have?

   b. Which words or phrases give you a clue to the funny meaning?

3. **Q.** What's the difference between a fish and a piano?
   A. You can tune a piano, but you can't tuna fish.

   a. Which word in the answer can be changed by separating the syllables?

   b. What does the word become?

   c. What is the meaning of the new words?

   d. Which words or phrases in the question give you a clue to the new words?

4. **Q.** Who is the best fencer in the ocean?
   A. The swordfish.

   a. What words can be formed by separating the syllables of a word in the answer?

   b. What is the meaning of the new words?

   c. Which words or phrases in the question give you a clue to the new words?

Activity

Stress and Pausing
Changes and Humor

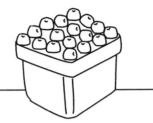

Directions

The meaning of a sentence can change if you change your stress and pausing. Sometimes these changes can make a sentence funny. Read each joke and answer the questions that follow.

1. "Knock-knock."   "Who's there?"   "Tennis."   "Tennis who?"   "Tennis more than nine."

   a. Which word in this joke can be changed by separating the syllables?

   b. What does the word become?

   c. Which words or phrases give you a clue to the new words?

2. **Q.** What are unhappy cranberries called?
   A. Blueberries.

   a. What words can be formed by separating the syllables of the word in the answer?

   b. What is the meaning of the new words?

   c. Which words or phrases in the question give you a clue to the new words?

3. **Q.** What do you call a witch who lives at the beach?
   A. Sandwich.

   a. What words can be formed by separating the syllables of the word in the answer?

   b. What is the meaning of the new words?

   c. Which words or phrases in the question give you a clue to the the new words?

4. Bestseller: *Early One Mornin'*
              by R. U. Upjohn

   a. What funny meaning can the author's name have?

   b. Which words or phrases give you a clue to the funny meaning?

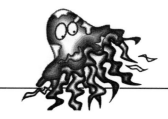

Stress and Pausing
Changes and Humor

Directions

The meaning of a sentence can change if you change your stress and pausing. Sometimes these changes can make a sentence funny. Read each joke and answer the questions that follow.

1. **Q.** What fish goes well with peanut butter in a sandwich?   **A.** Jellyfish.

   a. What words can be formed by separating the syllables of the word in the answer?

   b. What is the meaning of the new words?

   c. Which words or phrases in the question give you a clue to the new words?

2. **Shelby:** Did you hear about my friend Kerch?
   Molly: Kerch who?
   Shelby: Gesundheit!

   a. Which two words in this joke can be combined to form a new word?

   b. What is the new word?

   c. What does the new word mean?

   d. Which words or phrases give you a clue to the new word?

3. "Knock-knock."   "Who's there?"   "Norma."   "Norma who?"   "Norma Lee I don't tell knock-knock jokes."

   a. Which two words in this joke can be combined to form a new word?

   b. What is the new word?

   c. What does the new word mean?

4. Bestseller: *Living with Depression*
             by I. M. Blue

   a. What funny meaning can the author's name have?

   b. Which words or phrases give you a clue to the funny meaning?

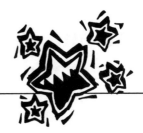

Activity

Stress and Pausing
Changes and Humor

Directions

The meaning of a sentence can change if you change your stress and pausing. Sometimes these changes can make a sentence funny. Read each joke and answer the questions that follow.

1. Bestseller: *Astrology—What the Stars Mean*
              by Horace Cope

   a. What funny meaning can the author's name have?

   b. Which words or phrases give you a clue to the funny meaning?

2. **Q.** Where do sharks come from?
   A. Finland.

   a. What words can be formed by separating the syllables of the word in the answer?

   b. What is the meaning of the new words?

   c. Which words or phrases in the question give you a clue to the new words?

3. **Q.** Who is the best-known mouse of all?
   A. Fay Mouse.

   a. What new word can be formed by combining the words in the answer and slightly changing the sounds?

   b. What does the new word mean?

   c. Which words or phrases in the question give you a clue to the new word?

4. **Q.** Where do snowflakes dance?
   A. At a snowball.

   a. What words can be formed by separating the syllables of a word in the answer?

   b. What is the meaning of the new words?

   c. Which words or phrases in the question give you a clue to the new words?

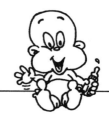

Stress and Pausing
Changes and Humor

Directions

The meaning of a sentence can change if you change your stress and pausing. Sometimes these changes can make a sentence funny. Read each joke and answer the questions that follow.

1. **Teacher:** Use *helpless* in a sentence.
   Max: Except for my baby brother, I helpless than anyone around the house.

   a. What words can be formed by separating the syllables of a word in the teacher's question?

   b. What is the meaning of the new words?

   c. Which words or phrases in Max's answer give you a clue to the new words?

2. **Q.** Who quit gymnastics because of poor balance?
   A. Eileen Wright.

   a. What words can be formed by separating the syllables of the first word in the answer?

   b. What is the meaning of the new words?

3. Bestseller: *Learn How to Mix Chemicals*
          by Yul B. Sari

   a. What funny meaning can the author's name have?

   b. Which words or phrases give you a clue to the funny meaning?

4. **Donald:** We found a duckway last night.
   Daisy: What's a duckway?
   Donald: Oh, about five pounds.

   a. What words can be formed by separating the syllables of a word in Daisy's question?

   b. What is the meaning of the new words?

   c. Which words or phrases in Donald's second comment give you a clue to the new words?

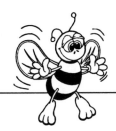

Activity

Stress and Pausing
Changes and Humor

Directions

The meaning of a sentence can change if you change your stress and pausing. Sometimes these changes can make a sentence funny. Read each joke and answer the questions that follow.

1. Bestseller: *How I Struck It Rich*
   by Jack Pot

   a. What funny meaning can the author's name have?

   b. Which words or phrases give you a clue to the funny meaning?

2. **Teacher:** Use the word *slogan* in a sentence.
   Arthur: The sheriff shot the bank robber first because the robber drew a slogan.

   a. What words can be formed by separating the syllables of a word in the teacher's question?

   b. What is the meaning of the new words?

   c. Which words or phrases in Arthur's comment give you a clue to the new words?

3. Movie: *Trapped in the Arctic*
   starring I. C. Waters

   a. What funny meaning can the movie star's name have?

   b. Which words or phrases give you a clue to the funny meaning?

4. **Q.** Why did little Jim put a bee on his knee?   **A.** He wanted to be a bee knee baby.

   a. Which two words in the answer can be combined to form a new word?

   b. What is the new word?

   c. What does the new word mean?

   d. Which words or phrases in the answer give you a clue to the new word?

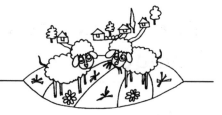

Stress and Pausing
Changes and Humor

Directions

The meaning of a sentence can change if you change your stress and pausing. Sometimes these changes can make a sentence funny. Read each joke and answer the questions that follow.

1. Movie: *Police Beat*
   starring Laura Norder

   a. What funny meaning can the movie star's name have?

   b. Which words or phrases give you a clue to the funny meaning?

2. **Q.** What is a metaphor?
   A. That's where sheep go to eat grass.

   a. What words can be formed by separating the syllables and slightly changing the sounds of a word in the question?

   b. What is the meaning of the new words?

   c. Which words or phrases in the answer give you a clue to the new words?

3. **Q.** Does the invisible man have any children?
   A. How could he—he's not apparent.

   a. What words can be formed by separating the syllables of a word in the answer?

   b. What is the meaning of the new words?

   c. Which words or phrases in the question give you a clue to the new words?

4. **Teacher:** Use the word *lilac* in a sentence.
   Marcie: My brother's a good kid, but he can lilac anything.

   a. What words can be formed by separating the syllables and slightly changing the sounds of a word in Marcie's comment?

   b. What is the meaning of the new words?

Activity

Stress and Pausing
Changes and Humor

Directions

The meaning of a sentence can change if you change your stress and pausing. Sometimes these changes can make a sentence funny. Read each joke and answer the questions that follow.

1. **Q.** What is a knob?   **A.** Just another thing to adore.

    a. What words can be formed by separating the syllables of a word in the answer?

    b. What does the original word mean?

    c. What is the meaning of the new words?

    d. Which words or phrases in the question give you a clue to the new words?

2. Movie: *Little Fish in a Big Pond*
            starring Ann Chovie

    a. What funny meaning can the movie star's name have?

    b. Which words or phrases give you a clue to the funny meaning?

3. "Knock-knock."   "Who's there?"   "Juicy."   "Juicy who?"   "Juicy the new video on MTV?"

    a. Which word in this joke can be separated and stressed differently to change its meaning?

    b. What phrase does the word become?

    c. Which words or phrases give you a clue to the new phrase?

4. A man walked up to the delivery window at the post office, where a new clerk was sorting mail. "Any mail for Mike Howe?" the man asked. The clerk ignored him, and the man repeated the question in a louder voice. Without looking up, the clerk replied, "No, none for your cow, and none for your horse either!"

    a. Which two words in this joke can be changed by moving the pause between the words and changing the stress?

    b. What do these words become?

    c. Which words or phrases give you a clue to the new words?

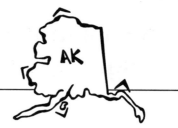

Activity

Stress and Pausing Changes and Humor

Directions

The meaning of a sentence can change if you change your stress and pausing. Sometimes these changes can make a sentence funny. Read each joke and answer the questions that follow.

1. **Teacher:** What is the capital of Alaska?
   Student: Juneau.
   Teacher: Of course I do, but I'm asking you.

   a. What words can be formed by separating the syllables and slightly changing the stress of the word in the student's response?

   b. What is the meaning of the new words?

   c. Which words or phrases give you a clue to the new words?

2. A girl camel with two humps married a boy camel with one hump. They had a baby with no humps. They named him Humphrey.

   a. What words can be formed by separating the syllables of a word in this joke?

   b. What is the meaning of the new words?

   c. Which words or phrases give you a clue to the new words?

3. Mrs. Clark decided she wanted to take a milk bath, so she asked the milkman for 10 gallons of milk. "Do you want it pasteurized?" the milkman asked. "No," replied Mrs. Clark, "up to my knees will be fine."

   a. What words can be formed by separating the syllables and slightly changing the sounds of a word in this joke?

   b. What is the meaning of the new words?

   c. Which words or phrases give you a clue to the new words?

4. **Q.** What did the scoutmaster say when his car horn was fixed?   **A.** Beep repaired.

   a. What new words can be formed by combining the sounds of the words in the answer in a different way?

   b. What do the new words mean?

   c. Which words or phrases in the question give you a clue to the new words?

Answer Key

Activity:
Stress and Pausing Changes and Humor

Page 159

1. (a) maybe so   (b) *Will He or Won't He*

2. (a) *two wrists*   (b) tourists   (c) *souvenirs*

Page 160

1. (a) *planet*   (b) plan it   (c) to think it out beforehand   (d) *Mars, Venus* (are planets)

2. (a) salamander   (b) *Reptiles*

3. (a) *tuna*   (b) tune a   (c) to adjust the musical pitch   (d) *piano*

4. (a) sword fish   (b) a fish who uses a sword   (c) *fencer, ocean*

Page 161

1. (a) *tennis*   (b) ten is   (c) *more than nine*

2. (a) blue berries   (b) sad berries   (c) *unhappy cranberries*

3. (a) sand witch   (b) a witch who lives at the beach   (c) *witch, beach*

4. (a) Are you up John?   (b) *Early One Mornin'*

Page 162

1. (a) jelly fish   (b) a fish made from fruit preserves   (c) *fish, goes well with peanut butter, sandwich*

2. (a) *Kerch who*   (b) kerchoo   (c) the sound someone makes when sneezing   (d) *gesund-heit* (something often said when someone sneezes)

3. (a) *Norma Lee*   (b) normally   (c) usually, under normal circumstances

4. (a) I am blue   (b) *Living with Depression*

Page 163

1. (a) horoscope   (b) *Astrology—What the Stars Mean*

2. (a) fin land   (b) a place where aquatic creatures that have fins live   (c) *sharks* (because they have fins)

3. (a) famous   (b) well-known   (c) *best-known*

4. (a) snow ball   (b) a dance for snow flakes   (c) *snowflakes, dance*

Page 164

1. (a) help less   (b) to assist with something in a minor way compared with others   (c) *baby brother, than anyone*

2. (a) I lean   (b) a person that tilts to one side

3. (a) you'll be sorry   (b) *Mix Chemicals* (because it can be dangerous)

4. (a) duck weigh   (b) the heaviness of a duck   (c) *five pounds*

Page 165

1. (a) jackpot   (b) *How I Struck It Rich*

2. (a) slow gun   (b) a sluggish firearm   (c) *the sheriff shot the bank robber first*

3. (a) icy waters   (b) *Arctic*

4. (a) *bee knee*   (b) beanie   (c) a small, stuffed animal   (d) *baby*

Page 166

1. (a) law and order   (b) *Police*

2. (a) meadow for   (b) a piece of grassy land   (c) *where sheep go to eat grass*

3. (a) a parent (b) a father or mother   (c) *have any children*

4. (a) lie like   (b) to tell untruths

Page 167

1. (a) a door   (b) to worship, to have loving admiration   (c) a barrier that can be opened or closed and generally has a knob   (d) _knob_

2. (a) anchovy   (b) _little fish_

3. (a) _juicy_   (b) did you see   (c) _new video on MTV_

4. (a) Mike Howe   (b) my cow   (c) _none for your cow, and none for your horse either_

Page 168

1. (a) do you know   (b) a question asking whether someone has knowledge or facts   (c) _of course I do, but I'm asking you_

2. (a) hump free   (b) having no humps (a rounded bump that sticks out)   (c) _camel, no humps_

3. (a) past your eyes   (b) higher than someone's eyes   (c) _bath, up to my knees will be fine_

4. (a) be prepared   (b) be ready for something   (c) _scoutmaster_

Unit 7:
Challenge Activities

Facilitator Information

Background

The development of metacognitive, metalinguistic, and metapragmatic skills required for true understanding of abstract language can best be achieved by exploring a wide range of language activities. Remember, there's more than one way to skin a cat!

Items that combine a number of elements of ambiguous language or humor are generally more difficult to explain than items based on one element. For example, the following item has both phoneme differences and stress and juncture changes that combine to create the humor.

Bestseller: Fighting Insomnia
by R. U. Upjohn and Eliza Wake

Visual items, such as solving word puzzles and drawing idioms and proverbs, provide yet another avenue to stimulate divergent thinking. These items can be more challenging to complete because they often rely on multistep cognitive processing (i.e., analyzing the visual cues, interpreting the representation, and explaining the meaning).

Knock-knock jokes offer excellent opportunities to facilitate an individual's understanding of phoneme differences, changes in stress and juncture, and, at times, a combination of the two. Some knock-knock jokes are based on dual interpretation of lexical items and comprehension of idiomatic expressions. For example:

"Knock-knock."   *"Who's there?"*   *"Hair."*   *"Hair who?"*   *"Hair today, gone tomorrow."*

The Activity in This Unit

This unit contains a variety of items, such as telling jokes, solving word puzzles, drawing idioms, completing idioms and proverbs, exploring metaphors and similes, and explaining knock-knock jokes. Tasks that target skills addressed in units 1–6, but that may likely present additional difficulties for individuals, also are presented.

The items in this unit provide numerous opportunities to enhance pragmatic skills as well. These opportunities arise as individuals:

1. Discuss the jokes and questions provided using think aloud and brainstorming techniques

2. Practice telling jokes

3. Practice paraphrasing messages to clarify meaning

4. Recognize a listener's inability to understand a message

5. Revise a message based on the listener's needs (e.g., simplifying the vocabulary when speaking to a younger person)

6. Provide appropriate repairs when communication breakdowns occur

Activity Presentation Suggestions

Since the items in this unit cover elements found in units 1–6, the ideas in the "Activity Presentation Suggestions" sections provided in those units would also apply to this unit. The tasks in this unit are often challenging for individuals and generally require the coordination of metacognitive, metalinguistic, and metapragmatic skills. The following ideas are specific suggestions for making activities more manageable for individuals:

- Use verbal mediation, brainstorming, and think aloud techniques to assist individuals with comprehending difficult tasks. For a description of each of these techniques, refer to pages 25–26.

- Discuss the meaning of the words *simile* (a figure of speech comparing two unlike items and usually containing the words *like* or *as*) and *metaphor* (a figure of speech in which a word or phrase that denotes one kind of object or idea is used in place of another to suggest a likeness between the items). Provide examples of similes and metaphors and encourage individuals to share examples of their own.

- Encourage individuals to develop their own knock-knock jokes (or to share ones they have heard elsewhere). Analyze these jokes by using questions similar to those found throughout this unit.

- Adjust the difficulty of a task by adding or removing variables. For example, a multiple-choice task can be made more difficult by removing the choices and requiring individuals to generate a response. Or, an explanation task can be simplified by having individuals respond to only some of the questions. Look for a variety of ways to increase or decrease the difficulty of tasks.

Activity

Unraveling Complex Language

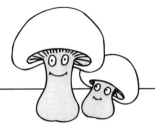

Directions

The following items target a variety of language skills. Complete each item.

1. _Joe was like a fish out of water._

   a. What do you think this simile means?

   - Joe was flopping around.
   - Joe was all dry.
   - Joe was feeling awkward and uncomfortable.

   b. Why might someone act like _a fish out of water?_

> _Simile—a comparison of two different things or ideas (usually contains the words_ like _or_ as)

2. **Tessa:** Jamal's answer was like music to my ears.

   a. What do you think Tessa's comment means?

   b. Select the most likely reason for Tessa's comment.

   - Jamal said Tessa got the lead in the school play.
   - Jamal was playing the flute.
   - Jamal said Tessa should have studied harder for her science test.

3. _Her head is a mushroom._

   a. What do you think this metaphor means?

   - She looks like a vegetable.
   - She has a bouffant hairstyle.
   - She has a headache.

   b. Explain your choice.

> _Metaphor—a word or a phrase used in place of another to suggest a likeness between two different things or ideas (does not contain the words_ like _or_ as)

4. _Her voice was cotton candy._

   a. What do you think this metaphor means?

   b. Now make a metaphor of your own.

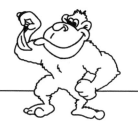

Activity

Unraveling
Complex Language

Directions

The following items target a variety of language skills. Complete each item.

1. Bestseller: *This House Is Haunted*
            by Les Gettaway and Hugo First

   a. What funny meaning can the authors' names have?

   b. Which words or phrases give you a clue to the funny meaning?

2.   Y
        R
        R
        U
        H

   > *Word puzzle—a visual display of a familiar expression*

   a. What statement is represented in the word puzzle above?

   b. Explain two possible meanings of the statement.

3. "Knock-knock." "Who's there?" "Gorilla." "Gorilla who?" "Gorilla cheese sandwich."

   a. How can you change the word *gorilla* to make sense of the final statement?

   b. Which words or phrases give you a clue for how to change the word?

4. A piece of rope went into a diner to get a soda. The waiter said, "We don't serve ropes here." Disappointed, the rope left the diner. A little while later, he had an idea. He stopped a man and said, "Will you please tie a knot in me and separate my strands at both ends?" Then he went back into the diner and ordered a soda. The waiter asked, "Say, aren't you the same rope who was in here before?" "No," said the rope, "I'm a frayed knot."

   a. What new words can be formed by combining the syllables of two words in the rope's final response?

   b. What is the meaning of the new words?

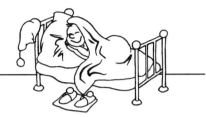

Activity

Unraveling Complex Language

Directions

The following items target a variety of language skills. Complete each item.

1.   **stay**   **me**

    a. What statement is represented in the word puzzle above?

    b. Explain two possible meanings of the statement.

> *Word puzzle—a visual display of a familiar expression*

2. **Q.** What's a diet?   **A.** A penalty for exceeding the feed limit.

    a. What familiar expression is changed to create this joke?

    b. What sound change is made to create this joke?

    c. Which words or phrases in the question give you a clue to why the sound change is made?

3. *The boys were animals as they rushed to be the first in line for lunch.*
    a. What do you think this metaphor means?

    - The boys were mad.
    - The boys ran and shoved each other as they got in line for lunch.
    - The boys were lazy and made rude noises.

    b. Explain your choice.

> *Metaphor—a word or a phrase used in place of another to suggest a likeness between two different things or ideas (does not contain the words* like *or* as*)*

4. Draw one or more of the following statements on a piece of paper. Present the drawing to another person, and ask him or her to guess the statement. Talk about two possible meanings of the statement.

    - I decided to catch some z's
    - Her name rings a bell
    - She stole the show

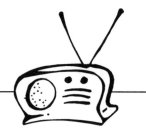

Activity

Unraveling
Complex Language

Directions

The following items target a variety of language skills. Complete each item.

1.   **EZ**

   iiiiiiiiiiiii

> *Word puzzle—a visual display of a familiar expression*

   a. What statement is represented in the word puzzle above?

   b. Explain two possible meanings of the statement.

2. **Peggy:** Does your radio work?   **Sue:** No, it plays.

   a. Which word in Peggy's question can have two meanings?

   b. What does Peggy mean?

   c. Which word in Sue's response can have two meanings?

   d. What does Sue mean?

3. Draw one or more of the following statements on a piece of paper. Present the drawing to another person, and ask him or her to guess the statement. Talk about two possible meanings of the statement.

   • Go fly a kite

   • Will you give me a hand

   • I was very angry, but I held my tongue

4. "Knock-knock." "Who's there?" "Jamaica." "Jamaica who?" "Jamaica mistake?"

   a. Which word can be separated and stressed differently to make this joke funny?

   b. What phrase does the word become?

Activity

Unraveling
Complex Language

Directions

The following items target a variety of language skills. Complete each item.

1. Create a knock-knock joke or a riddle about an animal. Tell the joke to someone else.

2. **Bess:** My sister fell down a flight of stairs last night and broke her leg.
    Jess: Cellar?
    Bess: No. My folks will still keep her around.

    a. Which word in this joke can be separated into two words?

    b. What does the word mean in Jess's question?

    c. What does Bess think Jess means?

    d. Which words or phrases give you a clue to each meaning?

3. **Q.** Do you know why the boy put his bed in the fireplace?
    A. He wanted to sleep like a log.

    a. What does the expression _sleep like a log_ mean?

    b. Give an example of another expression that means the same as _sleep like a log_.

4. **Q.** Why did the vet operate on the dog?   **A.** Because a stitch in time saves canine.

    a. Which phrase in the answer is based on a popular proverb?

    b. What is the proverb?

    c. Which syllable was added to change the phrase?

    d. Which words or phrases tell why the syllable was added to make this joke funny?

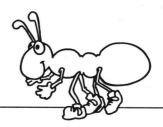

Activity

Unraveling Complex Language

Directions

The following items target a variety of language skills. Complete each item.

1. **Rich:** My boss has taken up the art of tumbling.
   Judy: Why did he do that?
   Rich: Because he has a gallbladder condition. He heard that a rolling boss gathers no stones.

   a. Which phrase in the last sentence is based on a well-known proverb?

   b. What is the proverb?

   c. What can the proverb mean?

2. A football coach saw his championship hopes fade when, with 10 seconds left in the game and his team behind by three points, a rookie player lost the ball. The other team picked it up and scored a touchdown. "Well," said the coach sadly, "that's the way the rookie fumbles."

   a. What familiar expression is the coach's comment based on?

   b. Which two words in the expression are changed to create this joke?

   c. Why are the words changed in this way?

3. Two ants wandered inside a large-screen TV set. After crawling around for hours, the first ant started to cry, "I think were lost!" "Don't worry, we'll get out," said the second ant confidently. "I brought along a *TV Guide.*"

   a. Which phrase in this joke can have two meanings?

   b. What does the ant mean when he uses the phrase?

   c. What else can the phrase mean?

4. Make a knock-knock joke using the name Ken.

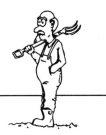

Activity

Unraveling Complex Language

Directions

The following items target a variety of language skills. Complete each item.

1.   **ECAP**

          PACE

> *Word puzzle—a visual display of a familiar expression*

   a. What statement is represented in the word puzzle above?

   b. Explain two possible meanings of the statement.

2. **Mother:** How do you like your new teacher?
   Little girl: I don't like her very much.
   Mother: Why not?
   Little girl: She told me to sit up front for the present, and then she didn't give it to me.

   a. Which word in the little girl's last comment can have two meanings?

   b. What does the teacher mean when she uses the word?

   c. What does the little girl think the teacher means?

   d. Which words or phrases give you a clue to the little girl's interpretation?

3. **Q.** Why did the farmer invite his two new hens to a party?
   A. He was trying to make hens meet.

   a. Which word is used to make this joke funny?

   b. What familiar expression is the answer based on?

   c. What does the expression mean?

4. **Q.** Why does time fly?   **A.** To get away from all the people who are trying to kill it.

   a. What two familiar expressions are the basis of the humor in this joke?

   b. What does each expression mean?

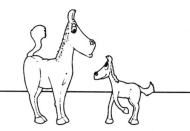

Activity

Unraveling Complex Language

Directions

The following items target a variety of language skills. Complete each item.

1. **Employer:** Where did you get your legal training?
   Applicant: Yale.
   Employer: You should be perfect for the job. What's your name?
   Applicant: Yohnson.

   a. Explain why this joke is funny.

   b. Which sound is changed to create the humor?

2. Talking Eyes: Our eyes often express our thoughts. Look at the eyes in the box. What do they seem to be saying?

   • "Which way did it go?"

   • "The moon is covered by clouds."

   • "I told you not to touch that!"

   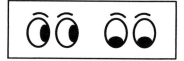

3. A young horse was talking with his mother. "Listen," he said, "compared to me, Man-o'-War was a nag. And as for Affirmed, when I grow up, I'll break every record he ever set!" "Son," sighed the mother, "you're living in a foal's paradise."
   a. What expression is this joke based on?

   b. What does the expression mean?

   c. Which word in the expression is changed in this joke?

   d. What is the word changed to?

   e. Why was it changed in this way?

4. **W O N A L I C E D E R L A N D**

   a. What childhood story title is shown in the word puzzle above?

   b. Explain the meaning of the way the words are arranged.

   > *Word puzzle—a visual display of a familiar expression*

Activity

Unraveling Complex Language

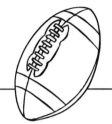

Directions

The following items target a variety of language skills. Complete each item.

1. **Lou:** What's a football made of?
   Bud: Pig's hide.
   Lou: Why should they hide?
   Bud: No. The pig's outside.
   Lou: Well, bring him in. Any friend of yours is a friend of mine.

   a. Which two words in this joke can each have two meanings?

   b. How does Lou interpret the words?

   c. What does Bud mean when he uses the words?

2. **Butcher:** The lamb I got in today is excellent.
   Butcher's wife: Must you always talk chop?

   a. What expression is the wife's comment based on?

   b. What does the expression mean?

   c. Which word in the wife's comment has a changed sound?

   d. Why was the sound change made in this way?

3. *From the window of the plane, the people below were like ants.*

   a. Which word in this statement describes people?

   b. Why are they being described in this way?

   > *Simile—a comparison of two different things or ideas (usually contains the words* like *or* as)

4. Review of a book about herbs: It's sage and thyme-ly.

   a. Which word in this review can be spelled differently to change its meaning?

   b. What does the word mean as it is spelled above?

   c. What does the word mean with its changed spelling?

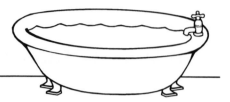

Activity

Unraveling Complex Language

Directions

The following items target a variety of language skills. Complete each item.

1. "Knock-knock." "Who's there?" "Dwayne." "Dwayne who?" "Dwayne the tub, I'm dwowning!"

   a. Which words have a sound change that make this joke funny?

   b. Create a knock-knock joke that has a sound change.

2. Mr. Oliver was proud of his ability to remember names. One afternoon, he met a neighbor who introduced him to her friend, Mary Hummock. "Hummock, hummock, rhymes with stomach," he thought. "Now I'll be sure to remember her name." Several days later, Mr. Oliver saw her again and smiled as he said, "Hello, nice to see you again, Mary Kelly."

   a. Why do you think Mr. Oliver called his neighbor's friend Mary Kelly instead of Mary Hummock?

   b. What do you do when you want to remember someone's name?

3. The father polar bear, the mother polar bear, and the baby polar bear were all sitting on a chilly iceberg. "I've got a tale to tell," said the father polar bear. Then the mother polar bear said, "And I've got a tale to tell too." Just then the baby polar bear stood up. "Brrrr! My tail is told!"

   a. Which phrase makes this joke funny?

   b. What does the baby polar bear really mean when she says "My tail is told!"?

   c. Which words or phrases give you a clue to the funny meaning?

4. Sign in an auto repair shop: "May we have the next _____?"

   a. What is the missing word in the sign above?

   b. Which words or phrases give you a clue to the missing word?

   c. What familiar expression is the sign based on?

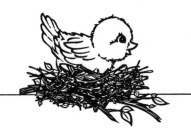

Unraveling Complex Language

Directions

The following items target a variety of language skills. Complete each item.

1. Once upon a time, there were two skunks named In and Out. When In was out, Out was in. When Out was out, In was in. One day, Out was in and In was out. Mother skunk, who was in with Out, said, "Out, I want you to go out and bring In in." And in two shakes of his tail, Out went out and brought In in. "How did you find In so quickly?" Mother skunk asked. "It was easy, instinct!"

   a. What does Out mean by *instinct*?

   b. What else could Out mean?

2. Talking Eyes: Our eyes often express our thoughts. Look at the eyes in the box. What do they seem to be saying?

   • "Do you have the time?"

   • "Don't move! It's crawling up your leg!"

   • "When are we going to the beach?"

   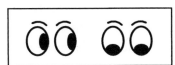

3. Bestseller: *Fighting Insomnia*
           by R. U. Upjohn and Eliza Wake

   a. What funny meanings can the authors' names have?

   b. Which words or phrases in this joke give you a clue to the funny meanings?

4. *Her hair was a nest.*

   a. Tell the meaning of the metaphor above.

   b. Create a metaphor that is similar to the one above.

> *Metaphor—a word or a phrase used in place of another to suggest a likeness between two different things or ideas (does not contain the words* like *or* as)

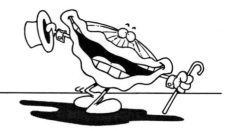

Unraveling Complex Language

Directions

The following items target a variety of language skills. Complete each item.

1.   **C**
      A
      L
      M

> *Word puzzle—a visual display of a familiar expression*

   a. What expression is represented in the word puzzle above?

   b. Explain two possible meanings of the expression.

2. Draw one or more of the following statements on a piece of paper. Present the drawing to another person, and ask him or her to guess the statement. Talk about two possible meanings of the statement.

   • My brother gets in my hair
   • He's on top of the world
   • He's a pain in the neck

3. Little Eddie visited the pet store with his father. Eddie watched two frisky kittens—Kate and Edith—playing in a cage. Eddie's father said he could choose a pet to purchase. Eddie chose Kate, but then begged to take Edith home too. Eddie's father replied, "You can't have your Kate and Edith too."

   a. What does Eddie's father mean?

   b. What familiar expression is Eddie's father's reply based on?

4. Sam the Clam ran a club that featured disco dancing. After leaving Sam's club, the harpist realized that she had forgotten her harp. "Oh no," she said, "I left my harp in Sam Clam's disco!"

   a. Which phrase in this joke sounds like the title of a familiar song?

   b. What is the actual song title?

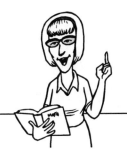

Activity

Unraveling
Complex Language

Directions

Fill in the missing letters to complete each familiar expression. Then explain the meaning of each expression.

1. Really good movies are f__w and f__r bet__ __ __n.

2. He started out on the __ __ __ng foot.

3. Her words went in one __a__ and out the o__ __ __ __.

4. She is so beautiful, she takes my br__ __ __ __ away.

5. My teacher says she has __y__ __ in the back of her head.

6. He jumped out of the f__ __ __ __ __ pan, into the __ __re.

Activity

Unraveling Complex Language

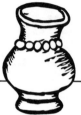

Directions

Fill in the missing letters to complete each familiar expression. Then explain the meaning of each expression.

1. I think I'm in h___ ___ ___ __t___ ___ because I broke the expensive vase.

2. If I were in his sh___ ___ ___, I would do the same thing.

3. You took too much food. Your eyes are ___ ___gg___ ___ than your __t___ ___ __ch.

4. P___ ___ ___ ___ ___ who live in ___ ___ ___ss houses should not throw stones.

5. He speaks with a forked t___ ___ ___ ___ ___.

6. Can't you sit still, or do you have ___ ___ ___s in your ___ __nt__?

Answer Key

Many responses in this unit will vary. The facilitator must judge the appropriateness of all responses. The answer key is merely meant to suggest some possibilities.

Activity: Unraveling Complex Language

Page 177

1. (a) *Joe was feeling awkward and uncomfortable.* (b) if he or she is in an unfamiliar place or situation

2. (a) Jamal's answer was very pleasant for her to hear (b) *Jamal said Tessa got the lead in the school play.*

3. (a) *She has a bouffant hairstyle.* (b) The head (or cap) of a mushroom is much wider than the stem. A bouffant hair style is wide.

4. (a) her voice was soft and sweet (b) her eyes were diamonds; his laugh was an alarm

Page 178

1. (a) *Les Getaway*—let's get away; *Hugo First*—you go first (b) *House, Haunted*

2. (a) hurry up (b) to go quickly; the letters that spell the word *hurry* are written going upward

3. (a) grill a (b) *cheese sandwich*

4. (a) afraid not (b) no, you are incorrect about that

Page 179

1. (a) Stay away from me (b) don't come near me; the word *stay* is set apart from the word *me*

2. (a) exceeding the speed limit (b) *sp* in *speed* was changed to *f* (c) *diet*

3. (a) *The boys ran and shoved each other as they got in line for lunch.* (b) hungry animals will often run and shove to get food, so that's how the boys were probably acting

4. Drawings will vary.

Page 180

1. (a) easy on the eyes   (b) something that (or someone who) is pleasant to look at; the letters *E* and *Z* are sitting on top of a row of *i*'s

2. (a) *work*   (b) is it operable; does it function?   (c) *plays*   (d) that the radio has fun instead of working

3. Drawings will vary.

4. (a) *Jamaica*   (b) did you make a

Page 181

1. Jokes will vary.

2. (a) *cellar* (b) the lowest level of a house; the basement   (c) sell her   (d) *flight of stairs, still keep her around*

3. (a) to sleep very deeply and soundly   (b) sleep like a baby; sleep like a rock

4. (a) *a stitch in time saves canine*   (b) a stitch in time saves nine   (c) *ca*   (d) *vet, dog* (which is a canine)

Page 182

1. (a) *a rolling boss gathers no stones*   (b) a rolling stone gathers no moss   (c) a person who keeps changing jobs or residences and accumulates no possessions or responsibilities; don't sit around if you want to get ahead in life; if you don't keep moving, you will miss out on life's adventures and challenges

2. (a) that's the way the cookie crumbles   (b) *cookie crumbles*   (c) *rookie fumbles*, which sounds like *cookie crumbles*, means the player with very little experience has dropped the ball

3. (a) *TV Guide*   (b) a plan or a map of the inside of a television set (c) the name of a magazine that shows the scheduled TV show lineup for a given week

4. "Knock-knock." "Who's there?" "Ken." "Ken who?" "Ken you hear me knocking on the door?"

Page 183

1. (a) pace back and forth   (b) to repeatedly walk for a short distance in one direction, then turn to walk back a short distance in the opposite direction; the word *pace* is first written backward and then written forward

2. (a) *present*   (b) for the time being   (c) a gift   (d) *she didn't give it to me*

3. (a) *hens*   (b) trying to make ends meet   (c) trying to live on a small amount of money

4. (a) *time flies; killing time*   (b) *time flies*—time goes by very quickly (especially when you're having fun); *killing time*—to waste time or to do something to make time pass

Page 184

1. (a) the applicant pronounced *jail* as *Yale* (the name of a prestigious university), so the employer was impressed with the applicant (even though he or she shouldn't have been)
   (b) *j* changed to *y*

2. *"Which way did it go?"*

3. (a) you're living in a fool's paradise   (b) to live under a condition of seeming happiness that is based on false assumptions and will not last; to deceive oneself   (c) *fool*   (d) *foal*
   (e) a *foal* is a young horse and *foal* sounds like *fool*

4. (a) *Alice in Wonderland*   (b) the name *Alice* appears in between the letters that spell the word *wonderland*

Page 185

1. (a) *hide, outside*   (b) *hide*—to remain out of sight, to screen from view; *outside*—outdoors
   (c) *hide*—the skin of an animal; *outside*—an animal's outside (hide)

2. (a) talk shop   (b) talk about things in your work or trade; talk about business matters at a social event (where business talk is out of place)   (c) *chop*   (d) because the man is a butcher, and he prepares and sells lamb chops

3. (a) *ants*   (b) they are seen from the window of a plane high above the ground, so they look very small

4. (a) *thyme-ly*   (b) the name of a garden herb   (c) appropriate or at just the right time

Page 186

1. (a) *Dwayne, dwowning*   (b) "Knock-knock." "Who's there?" "Baby owl." "Baby owl who?" "Baby owl see you later, baybe I won't."

2. (a) he switched the word *belly* for the word *stomach* in his memory trick   (b) repeat it as soon as you hear it; say it over and over to yourself; write it down

3. (a) *my tale is told!*   (b) my tail is cold   (c) *sitting on a chilly iceberg, tale to tell*

4. (a) *dents*   (b) *auto repair shop*   (c) May I have the next dance?

Page 187

1. (a) inner knowledge, awareness, or talent   (b) In has a bad smell

2. "Don't move! It's crawling up your leg!"

3. (a) Are You Up John? and He Lies Awake   (b) *Fighting Insomnia*

4. (a) her hair was messy   (b) her fingers were strings; his bedroom was a sty

Page 188

1. (a) calm down   (b) to become less excited; the letters that spell the word *calm* are written going downward

2. Drawings will vary.

3. (a) Eddie can't have both kittens   (b) you can't have your cake and eat it too

4. (a) *I left my harp in Sam Clam's disco*   (b) "I Left My Heart in San Francisco"

Page 189

1. *few* and *far* between
   not many; few and scattered; rare

2. started out on the *wrong* foot
   to have a bad beginning with a person or activity

3. in one *ear* and out the *other*
   to ignore; to not heed someone's advice

4. takes my *breath* away

   to surprise greatly; to impress very much; to leave speechless with surprise, wonder, or delight; to astonish

5. she has *eyes* in the back of her head

   to be able to sense what is going on outside of one's vision

6. out of the *frying* pan, into the *fire*

   to go from a bad situation to a worse situation

Page 190

1. in *hot water*

   in trouble

2. in his *shoes*

   seeing or experiencing something from someone else's point of view

3. your eyes are *bigger* than your *stomach*

   to take more food than one can eat

4. *people* who live in *glass* houses shouldn't throw stones

   do not complain about other people if you are as bad as they are

5. speaks with a forked *tongue*

   tells lies; tries to deceive others

6. have *ants* in your *pants*

   to be nervous, agitated, or excited

Appendices

Recording Form

NAME: _____

PRETEST DATE: _____   POSTTEST DATE: _____

ITEM TYPE	PREINTERVENTION PERFORMANCE (# OF CORRECT RESPONSES / # OF TASKS)		POSTINTERVENTION PERFORMANCE (# OF CORRECT RESPONSES / # OF TASKS)	
MULTIPLE-MEANING WORDS				
MULTIPLE-MEANING PHRASES				
MULTIPLE-MEANING SENTENCES				
SOUND CHANGES				
SWITCHING SOUNDS OR WORDS				
STRESS AND PAUSING CHANGES				
TOTALS				

COMMENTS:

Definitions of Idioms and Proverbs

The following is a list of definitions for the idioms and proverbs used in this resource (except those defined within the text of an activity). Other familiar idioms and proverbs are also included in this list to serve as a resource for creating additional tasks and game cards. The expressions are listed in alphabetical order.

a cat has nine lives—a cat can move so fast and jump so well that it seems to escape being killed many times

a chip off the old block—a person who behaves in the same way as a parent (usually the father) or resembles a parent

a face in the crowd—a person who blends in with the others in a group without making a noticeable impression

a fish out of water—a person who feels awkward and uncomfortable

a holdout—a rebel who refuses to go with the majority

a hole in one—an instance of succeeding on one's first try; a shot in golf that is hit from the tee and goes right into the cup

a horse of a different color—a person or object that is altogether separate and different

a rolling stone gathers no moss—a person who keeps changing jobs or residences and accumulates no possessions or responsibilities; don't sit around if you want to get ahead in life; if you don't keep moving, you will miss out on life's adventures and challenges

ace in the hole—someone or something important that is kept as a surprise until the right time so as to bring victory or success

agrees with—has a good effect on; suits

all in your mind—the way one feels, perceives, thinks, and reasons; a mental rather than an actual physical event

all right—well enough, correct, or suitable

all wet—mistaken, on the wrong track, or confused

all work and no play makes Jack a dull boy—one should have recreation as well as work to avoid becoming a boring person

an eye for an eye—every crime or injury should be punished or paid back as hard as it was inflicted

an open book—easy to understand completely

apple polishers—people who try to make others like them; people who try to win favor by flattery

back to square one—back to the beginning

back-seat driver—a bossy person in a car who always tells the driver what to do

beside the point—off the subject; about something different

blew his top—became very excited, angry, hysterical, or furious; lost his temper

blood runs cold—chilled or shivering from great fright or horror; terrified

break your neck—to do all you possibly can; to try your hardest

bring someone up—to raise and care for someone

bring to a head—to cause some activity to reach the point of culmination

burn your bridges—to make decisions that can't be changed in the future; to leave no way to escape

butter up—to try to get the favor or friendship of a person by flattery or pleasantness

calm and collected—in a state of repose and freedom from turmoil or agitation

can see right through someone—to understand and detect the true nature of someone; to realize the falseness of someone

can't have your cake and eat it too—you can't have it both ways; you can't both keep something and use it up

carry the banner—to support a cause or an ideal with obvious advocacy

cash in your chips—to die

catch some z's—to take a nap; to go to sleep

clear out—to get out of some place; to leave

close up shop—to stop some activity; to shut a store at the end of a day's business

come to the point—to get to the important part of something

come up in the world—to gain success, wealth, or importance in life

cool your heels—to wait

count off—to count aloud from one end of a line of individuals to the other, each person counting in turn

dead on your feet—too tired to do more; exhausted

dig up—to find or get someone or something with some effort

dirt cheap—extremely inexpensive

do or die—to do something or die trying; very eager and determined attitude *doesn't fit the bill*—isn't exactly right; not the thing that is needed

doesn't give a hoot—doesn't care

doesn't know the meaning of the word fear—doesn't have any fear; to be brave

don't bite the hand that feeds you—don't do harm to someone who does good things for you

don't have the guts—to lack courage

don't know whether you're coming or going—unable to think clearly; confused

don't let the cat out of the bag—don't tell about something that is supposed to be a secret

don't lie down on the job—don't do your job poorly or fail to do it at all

don't spill the beans—don't tell a secret to someone who is not supposed to know about it

down-to-earth—shows good sense; practical

draw a blank—to get no response; to find nothing

draw the line—to decide when a limit has been reached; to set a limit to what will be done

drawn and quartered—dealt with very severely; to execute someone in the barbaric medieval fashion of having him or her torn into four pieces by four horses tearing his or her body in four different directions

dress down—to scold harshly

drop right off—to go to sleep without any difficulty

eat like a bird—to eat very little

face the music—to receive punishment; to accept the unpleasant results of one's own actions

feather your nest—to use power and prestige to provide for yourself selfishly (said especially of politicians who use their offices to make money for themselves)

fed up—to be bored or disgusted with someone or something

feel like a new man—to feel healthy, vigorous, and well again after an illness or emotional upheaval

few and far between—not many; few and widely scattered; not often met or found

first things first—the most important things must be taken care of first

flies off the handle—to lose your temper; to get very angry

flip your lid—to lose your temper

fly-by-night—irresponsible, unreliable, or untrustworthy; set up to make a lot of money in a hurry and then move along so customers can't find you to complain about your poor work

for old time's sake—to do something for someone mainly because you knew the person in the past *for the present*—for now; for a while; temporarily

from hand to hand—from one person to a series of other people

from the ground up—from the beginning; entirely; completely

full of bull—talking nonsense

get a kick out of—to receive special pleasure from someone or something

get your point across—to convey the important details in a discussion

get the jump on—to get ahead of; to have the advantage over

get up and go—energetic enthusiasm; ambitious determination; pep; drive; push

give a cold shoulder—to ignore someone; to reject someone

give the willies—to cause someone to be uncomfortable, fearful, or nervous

glad rags—best clothes; clothes worn to parties or on special occasions

go ballistic—to become extremely upset

go down in history—to be remembered or recorded; to be remembered as historically important

go out of your way—to make an extra effort; to do more than usual

go to bed with the chickens—to go to bed very early; go to bed at sundown

go whole hog—to do everything possible; to be extravagant

going broke—to lose all your money, especially by taking a chance; to owe more than you can pay

gone off your rocker—to go crazy

got sick and tired of—felt a strong dislike for someone or something; felt annoyed; felt exasperated

growing pains—troubles when something new is beginning or growing; pains in children's legs supposed to be caused by changes in their bodies as they grow

had me in stitches—caused someone to laugh loud and hard, over and over

hang tough—to be firm and stick to your position

have a crush on someone—to have someone be the object of your infatuation

have a screw loose—to act silly or crazy; to act in a strange way; to be foolish

have a way of growing on you—to become increasingly acceptable or attractive

have ants in your pants—to become nervous and agitated

have dibs on—to reserve or claim something for oneself

have eyes in the back of your head—to seem to be able to sense what is going on outside of your vision *have guts*—to be brave enough to do something dangerous or difficult

have two strikes against you—to have things working against you; to be in a difficult situation; to be unlikely to succeed

head for the hills—to get far away in a hurry; to run away and hide

head out—to go or point away; to leave; to start out

heart in your mouth—a feeling of great fear or nervousness

heave to—to bring a ship to a stop

high-hat—treating others as inferior; acting above others

hit the hay—to go to bed

hold your own—to do as well as anyone else

hold out an olive branch—to offer to end a dispute and be friendly; to offer reconciliation

hold the stage—to be active in a group; to attract attention

horn in—to try to participate in something without an invitation or welcome

hurry up—to move very quickly; to be in a rush

I wouldn't send a dog out on a night like this—no person, nor any other creature, should be made to go outside during harsh weather conditions

if you play with fire, you might get burned—if you take a big risk or try something dangerous, you might get into trouble

in a bad frame of mind—in an unhappy mood

in a fog—mentally confused; not sure what is happening; not alert

in a hole—in a difficult position; in some trouble

in a nutshell—in a few words; briefly, without telling all about it

in clover—rich or successful; having a pleasant or easy life

in great measure—to a great extent; largely

in hot water—in trouble

in one ear and out the other—to ignore; to not heed someone's advice

in someone else's shoes—seeing or experiencing something from someone else's point of view

it has its good points—it has its positive aspects

it's about time—it's long overdue; it's almost too late

John Doe—a name used for an unknown person, especially in police and law business

John Q. Public—a name used informally for the average citizen

jump down someone's throat—to suddenly become very angry at someone; to scold severely or angrily

jump to a conclusion—to judge or decide something without having all the facts; to reach unwarranted conclusions

keep the ball rolling—to cause something that is in progress to continue

keep time—to show the right time; to keep the beat; to keep the same rhythm

keep your cool—to stay calm and undisturbed

kick off—to start, launch, or begin; to die

kick the bucket—to die

kick up a fuss—to make trouble; to make a disturbance

kill time—to waste time or do something that causes the time to pass more rapidly

knock it off—to cease doing something; to quit

knock off—to burglarize someone; to quit doing something

knock yourself out—to go to a great deal of trouble to do something

know on which side your bread is buttered—to have your own best interest in mind

laid-back—relaxed and unperplexed by difficulties

laugh off—to dismiss with a laugh as not important or not serious; to not take seriously

lay it on the line—to say something plainly so that there can be no doubt; to tell truthfully; to speak very firmly and directly about something

leave no stone unturned—to try in every way; to do everything possible

let bygones be bygones—to let the past be forgotten

let down easy—to refuse or say "No" to someone in a pleasant manner; to tell bad news about a refusal or disappointment in a kindly way

let off steam—to release excess energy or anger; to get rid of physical energy or strong feelings through activity

let the cat out of the bag—to tell something that is supposed to be a secret

light out—to run as fast as you can; to depart from somewhere as quickly as possible

like a bump on a log—someone who is unresponsive and immobile

little by little—slowly; a bit at a time

live from hand to mouth—to live on little money and spend it as fast as it comes in; to live without saving for the future; to have just enough

living beyond your means—to spend more money than you can afford

living in a fool's paradise—to live under a condition of seeming happiness that is based on false assumptions and will not last; to deceive oneself

look like a million dollars—to look wonderful

look like something the cat dragged in—to look bedraggled and worn

lord it over—to dominate someone; to direct and control someone

lose your temper—to lose control over your anger; to become angry

made a spectacle of yourself—made a public scene or disturbance; attracted unfavorable attention

make a killing—to have a great success, especially in making money

make a pit stop—to make a short stop somewhere

make good—to succeed at something

make up your mind—to choose what to do; to decide

make your bed and lie in it—to be responsible for what you have done and accept the bad results

man about town—a fashionable man who leads a sophisticated life

money to burn—to have a great deal of money, more than is needed

mum's the word—you must keep information a secret; keep silent; don't tell anyone

music to my ears—something you like to hear

never entered your head—never came to your mind or your consciousness

never give a sucker an even break—never treat fairly a person who can be easily cheated or deceived

nice guys always finish last—if you don't treat others in an inconsiderate, mean, or nasty manner, you won't get ahead

off center—not exactly in the center or middle

off the track—irrelevant and immaterial

on easy street—having enough money to live very comfortably; living in luxury

on pins and needles—worried and nervous; anxious

on the blink—faulty; malfunctioning; inoperative

on the fence—not able, or not wanting to choose; in doubt; undecided

on the level—honest; dependably open and fair

on the other hand—an alternate way of looking at things; an alternate possibility *out of bounds*—outside the boundaries of the playing area; not doing what is proper; outside the rules of good behavior

out of your element—not in a natural or comfortable situation

out of the frying pan, into the fire—to go from a bad situation to a worse situation

pack off—to send away; to dismiss abruptly

pain in the neck—an obnoxious or annoying person or event

partial to—having a weakness for; feeling favorable toward

pass up—to let something go by; to refuse

pay the piper—to face the results of your actions; to receive punishment for something

people who live in glass houses should not throw stones—do not complain about other people if you are as bad as they are

pick on someone—to make a habit of annoying or bothering someone; to do or say bad things to someone

piece of cake—easy

play the market—to try to make money on the stock market by buying and selling stocks

play up to someone—to try to gain someone's favor

play with fire—to take a great risk

plug away—to keep trying something

pop off—to make a wisecrack or smart-aleck remark

pull a fast one—to deceive, trick, or gain the advantage over someone unfairly

pull a few strings—to secretly use influence and power, especially with people in charge or with people who have important jobs, to do or get something; to make use of friends to gain your wishes

pull the wool over someone's eyes—to fool someone into thinking well of you; to deceive

pull yourself together—to become calm after being excited or disturbed

put an end to—to make something end; to stop an action

put forth—to produce; to send out

put your money where your mouth is—don't just talk about something, do it

race against time—to be in a great hurry to finish a given project by a specified deadline

rain or shine—no matter what the weather is, the activity or event will occur *raise Cain*—to be noisy; to cause trouble

raise the dough—to solicit money for a particular project

ran out of juice—to have no more energy or strength

read the riot act—to give someone a strong warning or scolding

riding for a fall—risking failure or an accident, usually due to overconfidence

right away—immediately; without delay

rise and shine—to get out of bed and be lively and energetic

round figures—close approximations

rub someone the wrong way—to make someone a little angry; to do something not liked by someone; to annoy, bother, or irritate someone

ruffle someone's feathers—to upset or annoy someone

rule the roost—to be the boss or manager, especially at home

run around—to go to different places for company and pleasure

see right through someone—to realize the falseness of someone or something; to understand the true nature of someone or something

shoot the breeze—to spend some time chatting; to talk

show off—to display nicely for people to see

sleep like a log—to sleep very deeply and soundly

sleep like a top—to sleep very deeply and soundly

snug as a bug in a rug—to be comfortable and cozy

speak with a forked tongue—to tell lies; to try to deceive someone

squeak through—to be successful but almost fail; to win by a small score

start out on the wrong foot—to have a bad beginning with a person or activity

step on it—to hurry up; to go faster

stick your nose into other people's business—to interfere with someone or something; to have an unwelcomed interest in; to be impolitely curious

stole the show—gave the best performance

stuck-up—acting as if other people are not as good as you are; conceited; snobbish

take a hard line—to be firm with someone

take a powder—to leave hurriedly; to run out or away; to desert

take down—to write or record what is said; to pull to pieces; to reduce the pride or spirit of someone; to be humble

take off your hat to—to give honor, praise, and respect to

take your breath away—to surprise greatly; to impress very much; to leave speechless with surprise,
wonder, or delight; to astonish

take your medicine—to accept the punishment or bad fortune that you deserve

take to task—to reprove or scold for a fault or error

talk shop—to talk about things in your work or trade; to talk about business matters at a social
event (where business talk is out of place)

talking point—something good about a person or thing that can be talked about in selling it

tell a thing or two—to scold; to express your anger

that'll be the day—that day will never come; that will never happen

the coast is clear—no enemy or danger is in sight

the last straw—the last small, additional burden or problem that causes everything to collapse

throw in your towel—to quit; to admit defeat

tickled pink—to be very pleased

time flies—time goes by very quickly (especially when you are having fun)

time flies when you are having fun—time passes very quickly when you're enjoying yourself

time to spare—over and above the amount of time needed

too big for tour britches—too haughty for your status or age; disdainfully proud

top dog—the head of any business or organization; the most influential or most prestigious person in an establishment

top-drawer—of the best or most important kind

trying to make ends meet—trying to live on a small amount of money

turn over a new leaf—to start again with the intention of doing better

up in the air—not settled; uncertain; undecided

use your head—use your intelligence; show common sense

where on earth have you been—where in fact, really

wouldn't touch it with a 10-foot pole—wouldn't get involved with someone or something under
any circumstances

working for chicken feed—working for a very small amount of money

your eyes are bigger than your stomach—to have a desire for more food than you could possibly eat

you're putting me on—to exaggerate; to tease; to act as if something were true; to play a joke on

Yellow Deck: Multiple-Meaning Words

1. **Q.** Why did the bald man put a rabbit on his head?

   A. He wanted a full head of hare.

   a. Which word in the answer is used to make this joke funny?

   b. What does it mean the way it is spelled above?

   c. How else can it be spelled and what would it mean?

   d. Which words or phrases in the question give you a clue to each meaning?

2. **Q.** What animal needs to be oiled?

   A. Mice, because they squeak.

   a. Which word in the answer can have two meanings?

   b. What does it mean here?

   c. What else can it mean?

   d. Which words or phrases give you a clue to each meaning?

3. **Q.** Who doesn't mind being interrupted in the middle of a sentence?

   A. A convict.

   a. Which word in the question can have two meanings?

   b. What does it mean here?

   c. What else can it mean?

   d. Which words or phrases give you a clue to the first meaning?

   ★

4. **Q.** Why are Boy Scouts so tired on the first day of April?

   A. Because they've just had a 31-day March.

   a. Which word in the answer can have two meanings?

   b. What does it mean here?

   c. What else can it mean?

   d. Which words or phrases give you a clue to each meaning?

5. **Q.** How did the dog's stomach feel after he ate a 20-pound bag of dog food?

   A. Fed up.

   a. What is one meaning the answer can have?

   b. What else can it mean?

6. **Q.** What is eight inches long and three inches wide, yet holds a whole foot?

   A. A shoe.

   a. Which word in the question can have two meanings?

   b. What does it mean here?

   c. What else can it mean?

   d. Which words or phrases give you a clue to the first meaning?

Yellow Deck: Multiple-Meaning Words—*Continued*

7. **Q.** What happened to Ray when he was eaten by a shark?

A. He became X-Ray.

a. Which word in the answer is used to make this joke funny?

b. What does it mean the way it is spelled above?

c. How else can it be spelled and what would it mean?

d. Which words or phrases in the question give you a clue to the second meaning?

8. **Q.** Did you hear about the two boas who got married?

A. They had a crush on each other.

a. Which word in the answer can have two meanings?

b. What does it mean here?

c. What else can it mean?

d. Which words or phrases give you a clue to one of the meanings?

9. **Q.** Where in the United States do you hear the most piano playing?

A. In the Florida Keys.

a. Which word in the answer can have two meanings?

b. What does it mean here?

c. What else can it mean?

d. Which words or phrases give you a clue to each meaning?

10. **Q.** What did one Martian say to the other as they approached Earth?

A. "You'll like this place. It has atmosphere."

a. Which word in the answer can have two meanings?

b. What does it mean here?

c. What else can it mean?

d. Which words or phrases give you a clue to each meaning?

★

11. **Q.** What happened to the racecar driver who ate watermelon?

A. He had to make a pit stop.

a. Which word in the answer can have two meanings?

b. What does it mean here?

c. What else can it mean?

d. Which words or phrases give you a clue to each meaning?

12. **Q.** Why did a timid Little Rock from Arkansas go to Colorado?

A. To visit his Boulder cousin.

a. Which word in the answer is used to make this joke funny?

b. What does it mean the way it is spelled above?

c. How else can it be spelled and what would it mean?

d. Which words or phrases in the question give you a clue to each meaning?

As Far as Words Go © 2002 C.C. Spector
Duplication permitted for educational use only.

Yellow Deck: Multiple-Meaning Words—*Continued*

13. **Q.** Why do sponges do a good job?

   A. Because they become absorbed in their work.

   a. Which word in the answer can have two meanings?

   b. What does it mean here?

   c. What else can it mean?

   d. Which words or phrases in the question give you a clue to one of the meanings?

14. **Q.** Why can't you trust a shark?

   A. There's something fishy about him.

   a. Which word in the answer can have two meanings?

   b. What does it mean here?

   c. What else can it mean?

   d. Which words or phrases in the question give you a clue to each meaning?

15. **Q.** How does ketchup feel when it's near a hamburger?

   A. It relishes every moment.

   a. Which word in the answer can have two meanings?

   b. What does it mean here?

   c. What else can it mean?

   d. Which words or phrases in the question give you a clue to each meaning? ★

16. **Q.** How did the little girl like her balloon ride?

   A. She found it an uplifting experience.

   a. Which word in the answer can have two meanings?

   b. What does it mean here?

   c. What else can it mean?

   d. Which words give you a clue to each meaning?

17. Mama firefly to her husband, commenting on their son: "He's bright for his age, isn't he?"

   a. Which word in this joke can have two meanings?

   b. What does it mean here?

   c. What else can it mean?

   d. Which words or phrases give you a clue to each meaning?

18. **Q.** What kind of dot dances?

   A. A polka dot.

   a. Which word in the answer can have two meanings?

   b. What does it mean here?

   c. What else can it mean?

   d. Which words or phrases in the joke give you a clue to the funny meaning?

Yellow Deck: Multiple-Meaning Words—*Continued*

19. A patient called his dentist for an appointment. "Not today," said the dentist. "I have 18 cavities to fill." He hung up the phone, picked up his golf bag, and departed.

    a. Which word in this joke can have two meanings?

    b. What does the dentist mean?

    c. What does the patient think the dentist means?

    d. Which words or phrases give you a clue to each meaning? ★

20. **Mac:** Did you hear about the undertaker who buried a body in the wrong place?

    Zack: That was a grave mistake.

    a. Which word in Zack's comment can have two meanings?

    b. What does it mean here?

    c. What else can it mean?

    d. Which words or phrases give you a clue to each meaning?

21. A baby bear was born at the zoo yesterday. The newspaper sent a cub reporter to cover the story.

    a. Which word in this joke can have two meanings?

    b. What does it mean here?

    c. What else can it mean?

    d. Which words or phrases give you a clue to each meaning?

22. **Q.** How can you make a strawberry shake?
    A. Take it to see a horror movie.

    a. Which word in the question can have two meanings?

    b. What does it mean here?

    c. What else can it mean?

    d. Which words or phrases give you a clue to each meaning?

23. **Fran:** My cousin swallowed a frog.
    Anne: Did it make him sick?
    Fran: Sick? He's liable to croak any minute!

    a. Which word in Fran's last comment can have two meanings?

    b. What does it mean here?

    c. What else can it mean?

    d. Which words or phrases give you a clue to each meaning?

24. **Q.** What does a mouse shed when he cries?
    A. Mouseketears.

    a. Which word in this joke is used to make this joke funny?

    b. What does it mean the way it is spelled above?

    c. How else can it be spelled and what would it mean?

    d. Which words or phrases give you a clue to each meaning?

Yellow Deck: Multiple-Meaning Words—*Continued*

25. **Q.** Who is the best contortionist in the world?

    A. A sailor. He can sit on his chest.

    a. Which word in the answer can have two meanings?

    b. What does it mean here?

    c. What else can it mean?

    d. Which words or phrases give you a clue to each meaning?

26. **Q.** What did the big candle say to the little candle?

    A. "You're pretty bright for a little fellow."

    a. Which word in the answer can have two meanings?

    b. What does it mean here?

    c. What else can it mean?

    d. Which words or phrases give you a clue to each meaning? ■

27. **Customer:** Is your water supply healthy?
    Waiter: Yes, sir. We use only well water.

    a. Which word in the waiter's answer can have two meanings?

    b. What does the waiter mean?

    c. What else could the word mean?

    d. Which words or phrases give you a clue to each meaning?

28. Many migrating birds view an empty birdhouse along the way as a cheep hotel.

    a. Which word in the answer is used to make this joke funny?

    b. What does it mean the way it is spelled above?

    c. How else can it be spelled and what would it mean?

    d. Which words or phrases give you a clue to each meaning?

29. **Q.** Why do dragons sleep during the day?
    A. So they can fight knights.

    a. Which word in the answer is used to make this joke funny?

    b. What does it mean the way it is spelled above?

    c. How else can it be spelled and what would it mean?

    d. Which words or phrases give you a clue to each meaning?

30. Definition of *coal:* a substance that goes to the buyer and the cellar

    a. Which word in this definition is used to make this joke funny?

    b. What does it mean the way it is spelled above?

    c. How else can it be spelled and what would it mean?

    d. Which words or phrases give you a clue to each meaning?

Green Deck: Multiple-Meaning Phrases

1. **Passenger:** Fourth floor, please.
   Elevator operator: Here you are, son.
   Passenger: How dare you call me son?
   You're not my father.
   Elevator operator: I brought you up, didn't I?

   a. Which phrase in the elevator operator's last comment can have two meanings?

   b. What are the two meanings?

   c. Which words or phrases give you a clue to each meaning?

2. **Q.** Why does a porcupine always win an argument?

   A. She knows how to get her points across.

   a. Which phrase in the answer can have two meanings?

   b. What are the two meanings?

   c. Which words or phrases in the question give you a clue to each meaning?

3. **Q.** What happened when Mary fell into a pile of feathers?

   A. She was tickled pink.

   a. Which phrase in the answer can have two meanings?

   b. What does it mean here?

   c. What else can it mean?

   d. Which words or phrases in the question give you a clue to the first meaning?

4. Definition of *braces:* putting your money where your mouth is

   a. Which phrase in this definition can have two meanings?

   b. What does it mean here?

   c. What else can it mean?

   d. Which words or phrases give you a clue to the first meaning?

   ★

5. My brother got fired because of illness and fatigue. His boss got sick and tired of him!

   a. Which phrase in this joke can have two meanings?

   b. What does it mean here?

   c. What else can it mean?

   d. Which words or phrases give you a clue to the first meaning?

6. "Good heavens, Mother!" cried Whistler when he saw her scrubbing the floor. "Have you gone off your rocker?"

   a. Which phrase in this joke can have two meanings?

   b. What does it mean here?

   c. What else can it mean?

   d. Which words or phrases give you a clue to the first meaning?

Green Deck: Multiple-Meaning Phrases—*Continued*

7. **Q.** What did the football say to the football player?

   A. "I get a kick out of you."

   a. Which phrase in the answer can have two meanings?

   b. What does it mean here?

   c. What else can it mean?

   d. Which words or phrases in the question give you a clue to the first meaning?

10. Two skeletons were in a closet. One said to the other, "If we had any guts, we'd get out of here."

   a. Which phrase in this joke can have two meanings?

   b. What are the two meanings?

   c. Which words or phrases give you a clue to each meaning?

8. Did you hear about the masseuse who got fired? It seems he rubbed his customers the wrong way.

   a. Which phrase in this joke can have two meanings?

   b. What does it mean here?

   c. What else can it mean?

   d. Which words or phrases give you a clue to each meaning?

   ■

11. Show me a pink-striped mare, and I'll show you a horse of a different color.

   a. Which phrase in this joke can have two meanings?

   b. What does it mean here?

   c. What else can it mean?

   d. Which words or phrases give you a clue to the first meaning?

   ★

9. Headaches are all in your mind.

   a. Which phrase in this joke can have two meanings?

   b. What are the two meanings?

12. Even though people don't like warts, they have a way of growing on you.

   a. Which phrase in this joke can have two meanings?

   b. What does it mean here?

   c. What else can it mean?

   d. Which words or phrases give you a clue to the first meaning?

   ★

Green Deck: Multiple-Meaning Phrases—*Continued*

13. Great gift idea: a 12-foot pole for people who wouldn't touch things with a 10-foot pole

    a. Which phrase in this joke can have two meanings?

    b. What does it mean here?

    c. What else can it mean?

16. **Paul:** I know a restaurant where we can eat dirt cheap.

    Matthew: Who wants to eat dirt?

    a. Which phrase in Paul's comment can have two meanings?

    b. What does Paul mean?

    c. What does Matthew think Paul means?

14. **Stephanie:** Boy was I in hot water last night.

    Tom: How come?

    Stephanie: I took a bath.

    a. Which phrase in Stephanie's first comment can have two meanings?

    b. What are the two meanings?

    c. Which words or phrases give you a clue to one of the meanings?

17. **Jayne:** I can't sleep. What should I do?

    Jonathan: Lie near the edge of the bed and you'll drop right off.

    a. Which phrase in Jonathan's response can have two meanings?

    b. What are the two meanings?

    c. Which words or phrases give you a clue to each meaning?

15. **Sarah:** Were you nervous about asking your boss for a raise?

    Michelle: No. I was calm and collected.

    a. Which phrase in Michelle's response can have two meanings?

    b. What does Michelle mean?

    c. What else can the phrase mean?

18. **Ryan:** You can't drive that nail into the wall with a hairbrush.

    Kelly: Really?

    Ryan: Of course not. Use your head.

    a. Which phrase in Ryan's second comment can have two meanings?

    b. What does Ryan mean?

    c. What else can the phrase mean?

Green Deck: Multiple-Meaning Phrases—*Continued*

19. Did you hear about the French horn player whose toupee fell into his instrument? He spent the rest of the concert blowing his top.

   a. Which phrase in this joke can have two meanings?

   b. What does it mean here?

   c. What else can it mean?

   d. Which words or phrases give you a clue to the first meaning?

22. The U.S. government reports that 30 million people are overweight. These, of course, are round figures.

   a. Which phrase in this joke can have two meanings?

   b. What does it mean here?

   c. What else can it mean?

   d. Which words or phrases give you a clue to each meaning?

   ■

20. **Marc:** I was operated on last week and I really enjoyed it.

   Anthony: How come?

   Marc: The doctor had me in stitches.

   a. Which phrase in Marc's last comment can have two meanings?

   b. What are the two meanings?

   c. Which words or phrases give you a clue to each meaning?

23. Dr. Jekyll has a new potion. One sip and you'll feel like a new man.

   a. Which phrase in this joke can have two meanings?

   b. What does it mean here?

   c. What else can it mean?

   d. Which words or phrases give you a clue to each meaning?

21. I know a lady who is very fond of arguing. She won't eat anything that agrees with her.

   a. Which phrase in this joke can have two meanings?

   b. What are the two meanings?

   c. Which words or phrases give you a clue to one of the meanings?

24. Even Mason and Dixon had to draw the line somewhere.

   a. Which phrase in this joke can have two meanings?

   b. What are the two meanings?

   c. What do you know about the Mason-Dixon Line?

   ★

Green Deck: Multiple-Meaning Phrases—*Continued*

25. **Farmer:** On my farm, we go to bed with the chickens.

    City boy: In the city, we sleep in our own beds.

    a. Which phrase in the farmer's comment can have two meanings?

    b. What does the farmer mean?

    c. What does the city boy think the farmer means?

28. Did you hear about the queen who threatened to hang the court jester if he didn't collect the morning mist in a bottle? It was a case of dew or die.

    a. Which phrase in this joke is based on a familiar expression?

    b. What does the phrase mean here?

    c. What is the real expression?

    d. Which does the real expression mean?

26. **Jan:** My mother thinks I'm too thin.

    Fran: What gives you that idea?

    Jan: She is always saying she can see right through me.

    a. Which phrase in this joke can have two meanings?

    b. What does Jan think her mother means?

    c. What else could Jan's mother mean?

29. When two egotists meet, it's an "I" for an "I."

    a. Which phrase in this joke is based on a familiar expression?

    b. What does the phrase mean here?

    c. What is the real expression?

    d. What does the real expression mean?

27. **Peter:** I woke up this morning feeling awful. My head was spinning and everything went around and around.

    Wendy: You must have slept like a top.

    a. Which phrase in Wendy's comment can have two meanings?

    b. What does it mean here?

    c. What else can it mean?

    d. Which words or phrases in Peter's comment give you a clue to the first meaning?

30. **Q.** Why is it easy to fool sheep?

    A. You can always pull the wool over their eyes.

    a. Which phrase in the answer can have two meanings?

    b. What are the two meanings?

    c. Which words or phrases in the question give you a clue to each meaning?

Red Deck: Multiple-Meaning Sentences

1. He ran his hand through his hair and pulled out a cigar.

   a. What are the two possible meanings of this sentence?

   b. Why is the intended meaning unclear?

4. **Juan:** Haven't I seen your face somewhere else?

   Carla: I don't think so. It's always been between my ears.

   a. What does Juan mean?

   b. What does Carla think Juan means?

2. **Little girl:** I'd like to buy a puppy, sir. How much do they cost?

   Store owner: Fifty dollars apiece.

   Little girl: How much does a whole one cost?

   a. What does the store owner mean?

   b. What does the little girl think the store owner means?

5. **Mary:** Did you meet your son at the airport?

   Lou: Oh, goodness no! I've known him for years.

   a. What does Mary mean?

   b. What does Lou think Mary means?

3. **Mr. Jones:** Can you give me a room and a bath?

   Hotel clerk: I can give you a room, but you'll have to take your own bath.

   a. What does Mr. Jones mean?

   b. What does the hotel clerk think Mr. Jones means?

6. **Charles:** I can sing "The Star-Spangled Banner" for hours.

   Richard: So what. I can sing the "Stars and Stripes Forever."

   a. What does Charles mean?

   b. What does Richard mean?

Red Deck: Multiple-Meaning Sentences—*Continued*

---

7. **Kim:** How much birdseed should you get for a quarter?

   Jim: None. Quarters don't eat birdseed.

   a. What does Kim mean?

   b. What does Jim think Kim means?

---

9. That crime carries an automatic penalty of 20 years in Alabama.

   a. What are the two possible meanings of this sentence?

   b. Why is the intended meaning unclear?

   ★

---

8. **Georgia:** Where were you born?

   Annie: England.

   Georgia: What part?

   Annie: All of me, silly.

   a. What does Georgia's second question mean?

   b. What does Annie think Georgia means?

---

10. **Lilly:** In Detroit, a man is hit by a car every five minutes.

    Willie: Boy, I'll bet he's pretty beat up.

    a. What does Lilly mean?

    b. What does Willie think Lilly means?

Red Deck: Switching Sounds or Words

11. **Q.** What is the difference between a marathon runner and a commuter?

    A. One trains to run and the other runs to trains.

    a. Which phrases in the answer have words that are switched?

    b. What does each phrase mean?

    c. Why is the switch made in this way?

14. **Q.** What is the difference between two sailors and two broken clocks?

    A. The sailors go to the seas and the clocks cease to go.

    a. Which phrases in the answer have words that are switched?

    b. What does each phrase mean?

12. **Q.** What is the difference between a boy who is late for dinner and a baseball hit over the fence?

    A. One runs for home and the other is a home run.

    a. Which phrases in the answer have words that are switched?

    b. What does each phrase mean?

    c. Why is the switch made in this way?

15. **Q.** What is the difference between a person who can hardly stand up and seven days?

    A. One is a weak one and the other is one week.

    a. Which words in the answer are switched?

    b. What does each phrase mean?

    c. Why is the switch made in this way?

13. **Q.** What's the difference between a motion picture and a ski resort?

    A. One has a cast of hundreds and the other has hundreds of casts.

    a. Which phrases in the answer have words that are switched?

    b. What does each phrase mean?

    c. Why is the switch made in this way?

16. **Q.** What is the difference between a man who is frozen to death and a Scotsman at the North Pole?

    A. One is killed with the cold, the other is cold with the kilt.

    a. Which phrases in the answer have words that are switched?

    b. What does each phrase mean?

Red Deck: Switching Sounds or Words—*Continued*

17. **Q.** What is the difference between a church bell and a pickpocket in a crowd?

    A. One peals from the steeple, and the other steals from the people.

    a. Which words in the answer have switched sounds?

    b. Which sounds are switched?

    c. Why is the switch made in this way?

18. Definition of an *environmentalist:* someone who believes the living owes him a world

    a. Which words in this definition are switched?

    b. What expression is this definition based on?

    c. What does the expression mean?

    d. Why are the words switched in this way?

19. **Q.** What's the difference between a coyote and a flea?

    A. One howls on the prairie, and the other prowls on the hairy.

    a. Which words in the answer have switched sounds?

    b. Which sounds are switched?

    c. Why are the sounds switched in this way?

20. **Q.** What's the difference between a New Yorker and a dentist?

    A. One roots for the Yanks and the other yanks for the roots.

    a. Which phrases in the answer have words that are switched?

    b. What does each phrase mean?

    c. Why is the switch made in this way?

Red Deck: Stress and Pausing Changes

21. **Q.** What did the termite say when he walked into the tavern?

    A. "Is the bar tender here?"

    a. Which two words in the answer can be combined to form a new word?

    b. What is the new word?

    c. What does the new word mean?

    d. What does the termite mean?

22. Conserve water or the country may go from one ex-stream to another.

    a. Which word in this joke can be combined to form a new word?

    b. What is the new word and what does it mean?

    c. What is meant by *ex-stream?*

23. **Q.** What do you call a very small mummy?
    A. A minimum.

    a. What words can be formed by separating the syllables of a word in the answer?

    b. What is the meaning of the new words?

    c. Which words or phrases in the question give you a clue to the new words?

24. **Q.** Could Christmas trees grow in Los Angeles?

    A. No, but Hollywood.

    a. What words can be formed by separating the syllables of a word in the answer?

    b. What is the meaning of the new words?

    c. Which words or phrases in the question give you a clue to the new words?

25. **Q.** What did the sad little girl say when her puppy ran away?

    A. "Doggone."

    a. What does the word in the answer mean?

    b. What words can be formed by separating the syllables of the word in the answer?

    c. Which words or phrases in the question give you a clue to the new words?

26. "Knock-knock."   "Who's there."
    "Annapolis."   "Annapolis who?"
    "Annapolis a fruit."

    a. What words can be formed by separating the syllables of a word in this joke?

    b. Which words or phrases give you a clue to the new words?

Red Deck: Stress and Pausing Changes—*Continued*

27. Bestseller: *Over the Cliff*
        by Hugo Furst

    a. What funny meaning can the author's name have?

    b. Which words or phrases give you a clue to the funny meaning?

    ■

28. **Q.** Why did the scientist disconnect his doorbell?

    A. He wanted to win the Nobel Prize.

    a. What words can be formed by separating the syllables of a word in the answer?

    b. Which words or phrases give you a clue to the new words?

29. "Knock-knock." "Who's there?" "Want." "Want who?" "Very good. Now try counting to three."

    a. Which two words in this joke can be changed by moving the pause between the words and changing the stress?

    b. What do these words become?

    c. Which words or phrases give you a clue to the new words?

    ★

30. **Q.** What's the difference between the law and an ice cube?

    A. One is justice and the other is just ice.

    a. Why is the word *justice* used?

    b. Why are the words *just ice* used?

Orange Deck: Sound Changes

1. Definition of *acupuncture*: a jab well done

    a. Which word makes this joke funny?

    b. What do you think the real word is?

    c. Which words or phrases gives you a clue to why the funny word is used?

    d. Explain why the funny word was used.

4. **Q.** What is the best way to carve wood?

    A. Whittle by whittle.

    a. Which word makes this joke funny?

    b. What do you think the real word is?

    c. Which words or phrases give you a clue to why the funny word is used?

    d. Explain why the funny word is used.

2. **Q.** What goes "snap, crackle, and squeak?"
    A. Mice Krispies.

    a. Which word makes this joke funny?

    b. What do you think the real word is?

    c. Which words or phrases give you a clue to why the funny word is used?

    d. Explain why the funny word is used.

5. **Q.** What type of party do mice like best?

    A. A mousecarade party.

    a. Which word makes this joke funny?

    b. What do you think the real word is?

    c. Which words or phrases give you a clue to why the funny word is used?

    d. Explain why the funny word is used.

3. **Q.** What's purple and thousands of miles long?
    A. The Grape Wall of China.

    a. Which word in the answer makes this joke funny?

    b. What do you think the real word is?

    c. Which words or phrases give you a clue to why the funny word is used?

    d. Explain why the funny word is used.

6. Definition of *gossip:* letting the chat out of the bag

    a. Which word makes this definition funny?

    b. What do you think the real word is?

    c. Which words or phrases give you a clue to why the funny word is used?

    d. Explain why the funny word is used.

★

Orange Deck: Sound Changes—*Continued*

7. **David:** Did you know there's a ghost sitting in that chair?

   Eric: Why can't I see it?

   David: Because the ghost is clear.

   a. Which word in David's last comment makes this joke funny?

   b. What do you think the real word is?

   c. Which words or phrases give you a clue to why the funny word is used?

   d. Explain why the funny word is to used.

8. **Q.** Who do big ships fear will push them around?

   A. Thug boats.

   a. Which word makes this joke funny?

   b. What do you think the real word is?

   c. Which words or phrases give you a clue to why the funny word is used?

   d. Explain why the funny word is used.

9. **Q.** What do you call a fast dinosaur?

   A. A pronto-saurus.

   a. Which word makes this joke funny?

   b. What do you think the real word is?

   c. Which words or phrases give you a clue to why the funny word is used?

   d. Explain why the funny word is used.

10. **Q.** What game do little fish play?

    A. Salmon Says.

    a. Which word makes this joke funny?

    b. What do you think the real word is?

    c. Which words or phrases give you a clue to why the funny word is used?

    d. Explain why the funny word is used.

11. **Q.** What does a fencing master do at noon?

    A. He goes to lunge.

    a. Which word makes this joke funny?

    b. What do you think the real word is?

    c. Which words or phrases give you a clue to why the funny word is used?

    d. Explain why the funny word is used.

12. **Q.** What magazine do cats read?

    A. Good Mousekeeping.

    a. Which word makes this joke funny?

    b. What do you think the real word is?

    c. Which words or phrases give you a clue to why the funny word is used?

    d. Explain why the funny word is used.

Orange Deck: Sound Changes—*Continued*

13. **Q.** What is another name for a smart duck?

    A. A wise quacker.

    a. Which word makes this joke funny?

    b. What do you think the real word is?

    c. Which words or phrases give you a clue to why the funny word is used?

    d. Explain why the funny word is used.

16. Musical comedy about a gorilla:

    The Kong and I

    a. Which word makes this joke funny?

    b. What do you think the real word is?

    c. Which words or phrases give you a clue to why the funny word is used?

    d. Explain why the funny word is used.

    ★

14. **Baby candle:** Mama, I feel hot.

    Mama candle: Hush, dear, it's only glow-ing pains.

    a. Which word makes this joke funny?

    b. What do you think the real word is?

    c. Which words or phrases give you a clue to why the funny word is used?

    d. Explain why the funny word is used.

    ★

17. The mother snake gave birth to a bouncing baby boa.

    a. Which word makes this joke funny?

    b. What do you think the real word is?

    c. Which words or phrases give you a clue to why the funny word is used?

    d. Explain why the funny word is used.

15. **Q.** What do baby cats wear?

    A. Diapurrs.

    a. Which word makes this joke funny?

    b. What do you think the real word is?

    c. Which words or phrases give you a clue to why the funny word is used?

    d. Explain why the funny word is used.

18. There's a health-food store on Wall Street. It's for stocky brokers.

    a. Which word makes this joke funny?

    b. What do you think the real word is?

    c. Which words or phrases give you a clue to why the funny word is used?

    d. Explain why the funny word is used.

    ■

Orange Deck: Sound Changes—*Continued*

19. **Q.** What's a cat's favorite play?

    A. Ro-meow and Juliet.

    a. Which word makes this joke funny?

    b. What do you think the real word is?

    c. Which words or phrases give you a clue to why the funny word is used?

    d. Explain why the funny word is used.

20. **Q.** What is a dog's favorite car?

    A. A Hounda.

    a. Which word makes the joke funny?

    b. What do you think the real word is?

    c. Which words or phrases give you a clue to why the funny word is used?

    d. Explain why the funny word is used.

21. **Q.** Are cats rich?

    A. No, most are purr.

    a. Which word makes the joke funny?

    b. What do you think the real word is?

    c. Which words or phrases give you a clue to why the funny word is used?

    d. Explain why the funny word is used.

22. I know a man who calls his prize-winning dog a show-arf.

    a. Which word makes this joke funny?

    b. What do you think the real word is?

    c. Which words or phrases give you a clue to why the funny word is used?

    d. Explain why the funny word is used.

23. **Q.** What is a tiny hippo called?

    A. A hippopotamouse.

    a. Which word makes this joke funny?

    b. What do you think the real word is?

    c. Which words or phrases give you a clue to why the funny word is used?

    d. Explain why the funny word is used.

24. The Thunder God went for a ride on his favorite filly. "I'm Thor!" he cried. His horse replied, "Of course you're thore, you forgot the thaddle, thilly."

    a. Which words make this joke funny?

    b. What do you think the real words are?

    c. Which words or phrases give you a clue to why the funny words are used?

    d. Explain why the funny words are used.

Orange Deck: Sound Changes—*Continued*

25. **Q.** What could you bake for a police officer on her birthday?

    A. A copcake.

    a. Which word makes this joke funny?

    b. What do you think the real word is?

    c. Which words or phrases give you a clue to why the funny word is used?

    d. Explain why the funny word is used.

28. **Q.** Which apes like lemon pie?

    A. Meringue-utans.

    a. Which word makes this joke funny?

    b. What do you think the real word is?

    c. Which words or phrases give you a clue to why the funny word is used?

    d. Explain why the funny word is used.

26. **Q.** What do friendly cats say to each other?

    A. "Have a mice day!"

    a. Which word makes this joke funny?

    b. What do you think the real word is?

    c. Which words or phrases give you a clue to why the funny word is used?

    d. Explain why the funny word is used.

29. **Q.** What do you call a large white whale who can't make up his mind?

    A. Maybe Dick.

    a. Which word makes this joke funny?

    b. What do you think the real word is?

    c. Which words or phrases give you a clue to why the funny word is used?

    d. Explain why the funny word is used.

27. A best-selling novel could be described as "a plot of gold."

    a. Which word makes this joke funny?

    b. What do you think the real word is?

    c. Which words or phrases give you a clue to why the funny word is used?

    d. Explain why the funny word is used.

    ★

30. **Q.** What do outlaws eat for dessert?

    A. Crookies.

    a. Which word makes this joke funny?

    b. What do you think the real word is?

    c. Which words or phrases give you a clue to why the funny word is used?

    d. Explain why the funny word is used.

Blue Deck: Challenge Activities

1. *Helen's eyes were brimming pools.*

   a. Which phrase in this metaphor tells you about Helen's eyes?

   b. What do you think the phrase really means?

2. *Maggie was proud as a peacock.*

   a. Which phrase in this simile describes Maggie?

   b. What do you think the phrase really means?

3. *Tara is an open book.*

   a. Which phrase in this metaphor describes Tara?

   b. What do you think the phrase really means?

4. **Don:** Beth eats like a bird.

   Daphne: Yes, a vulture!

   a. Which phrase in this joke can have two meanings?

   b. What does Don mean?

   c. What does Daphne mean?

5. Talking Eyes: Our eyes often express our thoughts. Look at the eyes in the box. What do they seem to be saying?

   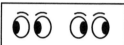

   - "I bought a new shirt."
   - "The cat wants to come inside."
   - "Psst! Can you keep a secret?"

6. Draw one or more of the following expressions on a piece of paper. Present the drawing to another person, and ask him or her to explain two possible meanings of the expression.

   - Butter him up
   - Knock it off
   - Back-seat driver

Blue Deck: Challenge Activities—*Continued*

7. C R ☺ W D

   a. What statement is represented in the word puzzle above?

   b. Explain two possible meanings of the statement.

---

8. Definition of *octopus*: a cat that lost one of its lives

   a. What familiar expression is this definition based on?

   b. Why is this expression used to define octopus?

---

9. *Arthur's feet were blocks of ice.*

   a. Which phrase in this metaphor describes Arthur's feet?

   b. What do you think the metaphor means?

---

10. Did you hear about the camper who backed into the campfire? He burned his britches.

   a. What familiar expression is this joke based on?

   b. What does the expression mean?

   c. How is the expression changed?

   d. Why is it changed in this way?

---

11. If you pl __ __ with f __ __ __, you may get burned.

   a. Fill in the missing letters to complete the expression above.

   b. Explain the meaning of this expression.

---

12. *Maggie was like a bump on a log.*

   a. What do you think this simile means?

   b. Why might someone be *a bump on a log?*

Blue Deck: Challenge Activities—*Continued*

13. Draw one or more of the following expressions on a piece of paper. Present the drawing to another person, and ask him or her to explain two possible meanings of the expression.

    • Keep your eye on the baby

    • Her name rings a bell

    • Pull yourself together

16. **parked parked**

    a. What statement is represented in the word puzzle above?

    b. Explain two possible meanings of the statement.

14. **n e PAIN c k**

    a. What statement is represented in the word puzzle above?

    b. Explain two possible meanings of the statement.

17. **my you're way**

    a. What statement is represented in the word puzzle above?

    b. Explain two possible meanings of the statement.

15. *The cat's fur was like a piece of black silk.*

    a. What do you think this simile means?

    b. Create a new simile about an animal.

18. *Jake was a popsicle stick.*

    a. Which words in this metaphor describe Jake?

    b. What do you think the words really mean?

Blue Deck: Challenge Activities—*Continued*

19. Sign in a florist shop: "Light up your garden. Plant a _____."

    a. What is the missing word in the sign above?

    b. Which words or phrases give you a clue to the missing word?

22. Bestseller: *Hopelessly Lost* by R.U. Sure and Wareham I. Now

    a. What funny meanings can the authors' names have?

    b. Which words or phrases give you a clue to the funny meanings?

20. Definition of a *flood*: a river that's too big for its bridges

    a. What familiar expression is this definition based on?

    b. What does the expression mean?

23. Draw one of the following expressions on a piece of paper. Present the drawing to another person, and ask him or her to explain two possible meanings of the statement.

    • Drove her crazy

    • Looking for trouble

    • Reach for the stars

21. **Connie:** You must have won the lottery.

    Jean: What makes you say that?

    Connie: You look like a million bucks.

    a. Which phrase in this joke can have two meanings?

    b. What are the two meanings?

24. Theo looked like something the cat dragged in.

    a. What do you think this simile means?

    b. Create another simile that describes how someone looks.

Blue Deck: Challenge Activities—*Continued*

25. **Danny:** Why are you wearing only one glove?

    Michael: The weather forecast said it might be warm today, but on the other hand, it might be cold.

    a. Which phrase in Michael's answer can have two meanings?

    b. What does Michael think the phrase means?

    c. What does it really mean?

28. **call   you   come**

    a. What statement is represented in the word puzzle above?

    b. Explain two possible meanings of the statement.

26. **Q.** What has a foot at each end and one in the middle?

    a. Which word in the question can have two meanings?

    b. What are the two meanings?

    c. What is the answer to this joke?

29. "Knock-knock." "Who's there?" "Gillette." "Gillette who?" "Gillette the cat out?"

    a. How can you change the word *Gillette* to cause the humor in this joke?

    b. Which words or phrases give you a clue to the new words?

27. Tell a knock-knock joke using the name Betty.

30. **Dan:** Is it bad luck to be followed by a cat?

    Ann: That depends. Are you a man or a mouse?

    a. Which phrase in Ann's answer can have two meanings?

    b. What does it mean here?

    c. What else can it mean?

Game Card Template

Game Cards Answer Key
Yellow Deck

Multiple-Meaning Words

1. (a) *hare*   (b) a rabbit   (c) hair—the covering that grows on your head   (d) *bald, rabbit, head*

2. (a) *squeak*   (b) a sharp cry or sound   (c) the sound a mouse makes   (d) *needs to be oiled, mice*

3. (a) *sentence*   (b) judgment stating the amount of time that must be served in prison   (c) a syntactic unit that expresses an assertion, question, or command   (d) *convict*

4. (a) *March*   (b) move along steadily, usually with a rhythmic stride and in step with others   (c) a month of the year   (d) *Boy Scouts so tired, April*

5. (a) full of food   (b) bored or disgusted with someone or something

6. (a) *foot*   (b) the end part of a leg on which people stand   (c) a unit of measurement twelve inches long   (d) *inches, shoe*

7. (a) *X-Ray*   (b) a method of examining, treating, or photographing the inside of a person or thing   (c) ex-Ray—the former Ray (he no longer exists)   (d) *eaten by a shark*

8. (a) *crush*   (b) the objects of infatuation   (c) to squeeze together with great force   (d) *boa*

9. (a) *Keys*   (b) a group of coral islets off the southern coast of Florida   (c) the levers of a keyboard musical instrument that produce tones   (d) *where in the United States, piano, Florida*

10. (a) *atmosphere*   (b) a feeling or mood associated with a particular place   (c) the whole mass of air surrounding the earth   (d) *Martian, Earth, you'll like this place*

11. (a) *pit*   (b) the seeds (pits) of the watermelon   (c) an area alongside an auto racecourse used for refueling and repairing the cars during a race; a short stop somewhere   (d) *racecar driver, ate watermelon, stop*

12. (a) *Boulder*   (b) a city in Colorado; a large rounded mass of rock   (c) *bolder*—fearless before danger; a daring spirit; assured; confident   (d) *timid, Little Rock, Arkansas, Colorado*

13. (a) *absorbed*   (b) become totally engrossed or engaged in an activity   (c) to suck up or take up water or other liquid   (d) *sponges*

14. (a) *fishy*   (b) creating doubt or suspicion; questionable   (c) smells like fish   (d) *can't trust, shark*

15. (a) *relishes*   (b) enjoyment or delight in something that satisfies your tastes or desires   (c) condiments (e.g., pickles or chopped onions) eaten with other foods to enhance their flavor   (d) *how does ketchup feel, hamburger*

16. (a) *uplifting*   (b) an improvement in one's spiritual, social, or intellectual condition   (c) to be lifted up in the air   (d) *like, balloon ride, experience*

17. (a) *bright*   (b) smart; intelligent   (c) radiating or reflecting light   (d) *mama firefly to her husband, their son, for his age*

18. (a) *polka*   (b) a dot in a pattern of regularly distributed dots   (c) a kind of dance; a lively Bohemian dance in 2/4 time   (d) *dances*

19. (a) *cavities*   (b) holes (on a golf course)   (c) areas of decay in teeth   (d) *patient, dentist, 18, golf bag*

20. (a) *grave*   (b) deserves serious consideration   (c) an excavation for burial of a body   (d) *undertaker, buried a body, wrong place, mistake*

21. (a) *cub*   (b) an inexperienced newspaper reporter   (c) a young bear   (d) *baby bear, newspaper, reporter*

22. (a) *shake*   (b) to tremble with fear   (c) a beverage usually made with milk and ice cream   (d) *strawberry, horror movie*

23. (a) *croak*   (b) to die   (c) the harsh sound a frog makes   (d) *frog, sick*

24. (a) *Mouseketears*   (b) tears shed by a mouse   (c) Musketeers—soldiers armed with muskets   (d) *mouse, cries*

25. (a) *chest*   (b) a part of the body enclosed by the ribs and breastbone   (c) a container for storage or shipping   (d) *contortionist, sailor*

26. (a) *bright*   (b) radiating and reflecting light   (c) smart; intelligent   (d) *candle, little fellow*

27. (a) *well*   (b) a hole sunk into the earth to reach a supply of water   (c) in good health   (d) *water supply healthy*

28. (a) *cheep*   (b) the sound made by a bird   (c) cheap—inexpensive   (d) *migrating birds, birdhouse, hotel*

29. (a) *knights*   (b) a medieval man at arms   (c) *nights*—the time from dusk to dawn when no sunlight is visible   (d) *dragons, sleep during the day, fight*

30. (a) *cellar*   (b) *lowest level of a house; the basement*   (c) seller—one that offers something for sale   (d) *coal, buyer*

Green Deck

Multiple-Meaning Phrases

1. (a) *brought you up*   (b) took you in the elevator from a lower floor to a higher one; raised you and took care of you   (c) *fourth floor, son, father*

2. (a) *get her points across*   (b) knows how to use the bristles that cover her body; knows how to tell the important details in a discussion   (c) *porcupine, win an argument*

3. (a) *tickled pink*   (b) tickled all over and turned pink   (c) was very pleased   (d) *pile of feathers*

4. (a) *putting your money where your mouth is*   (b) paying a large sum of money for braces on your teeth   (c) don't just talk about something, do it   (d) *braces*

5. (a) *got sick and tired of him*   (b) felt strong dislike for him; was annoyed; was exasperated   (c) his boss fired him because he was ill and fatigued   (d) *got fired*

6. (a) *gone off your rocker*   (b) gotten off a rocking chair   (c) gone crazy   (d) *Whistler* (man who painted a famous picture of his mother sitting in a rocking chair)

7. (a) *get a kick out of you*   (b) the football player gave the football a forceful thrust with his foot   (c) to receive special pleasure from someone   (d) *football, football player*

8. (a) *rubbed his customers the wrong way*   (b) moved his hands in a manner that was wrong when giving a massage   (c) to make someone a little angry; to do something not liked by someone; to annoy, bother, or irritate someone   (d) *masseuse, got fired*

9. (a) *all in your mind*   (b) inside your head; the way one feels, perceives, thinks, and reasons or a mental rather than an actual physical event

10. (a) *had any guts*   (b) had any insides, inner organs; to be brave enough to do something dangerous or difficult   (c) *skeletons, get out of here*

11. (a) *a horse of a different color*   (b) a horse that has pink stripes   (c) something altogether separate and different   (d) *pink-striped mare*

12. (a) *have a way of growing on you*   (b) they grow on your skin whether you want them or not   (c) become increasingly acceptable or attractive   (d) *warts*

13. (a) *wouldn't touch things with a 10-foot pole*   (b) would touch something if they had a pole longer than ten feet   (c) would not get involved with someone or something under any circumstances

14. (a) *in hot water*   (b) in a bathtub filled with hot water; in trouble   (c) *bath*

15. (a) *calm and collected*   (b) stayed calm and got a raise   (c) in a state of repose and freedom from turmoil or agitation

16. (a) *dirt cheap*   (b) extremely inexpensive food   (c) dirt is sold as inexpensive food

17. (a) *drop right off*   (b) fall off the edge of the bed; go to sleep without any difficulty   (c) *sleep, edge of the bed*

18. (a) *use your head*   (b) use your intelligence; show common sense   (c) use your head like a hammer to drive the nail into the wall

19. (a) *blowing his top*   (b) he blew his French horn with the toupee in it, so what was on top of his head was blown   (c) became very excited, angry, hysterical, or furious; lost his temper   (d) *toupee fell into his instrument*

20. (a) *had me in stitches*   (b) had stitches (i.e., sutures) as a result of a surgical procedure; caused someone to laugh loud and hard, over and over   (c) *operated on, I really enjoyed it, doctor*

21. (a) *agrees with her*   (b) the food has the same views and opinions as the lady; the food has a good effect on her or suits her   (c) *fond of arguing, won't eat*

22. (a) *round figures*   (b) close approximations   (c) sometimes a person who is overweight might have a rounder body figure   (d) *30 million, overweight*

23. (a) *feel like a new man*   (b) feel like a different person   (c) to feel healthy, vigorous, and well again after an illness or emotional upheaval   (d) *Dr. Jekyll, potion*

24. (a) *draw the line*   (b) physically draw a line between two things; to decide when a limit has been reached or to set a limit to what will be done   (c) a line that was drawn on a map of the United States that separated the north from the south before the Civil War

25. (a) *go to bed with the chickens*   (b) to go to bed very early; to go to bed at sundown   (c) to sleep in the same bed with the chickens

26. (a) *can see right through me*   (b) she's so thin her mother can see through her body   (c) to understand and detect the true nature of her; to realize the falseness of her

27. (a) *slept like a top*   (b) his head was going around and around like a spinning top   (c) to sleep very deeply and soundly   (d) *my head was spinning, everything went around and around*

28. (a) *dew or die*   (b) collect the morning dew or be hanged   (c) do or die   (d) to do something or die trying; to be very eager and determined

29. (a) *an "I" for an "I"*   (b) both people (e.g., the egotists) will be using the word "I" when they meet and talk since egotists like to talk about themselves   (c) an eye for an eye   (d) every crime or injury should be punished or paid back as hard as it is was inflicted

30. (a) *pull the wool over their eyes*   (b) to pull the wool on the sheeps' heads down over their eyes; to fool someone into thinking well of you or to deceive someone   (c) *fool sheep*

Red Deck

Multiple-Meaning Sentences

1. (a) he pulled a cigar out of his hair; he ran his hand through his hair, and then he pulled a cigar out of his pocket   (b) the words "then he" are implied but not stated

2. (a) it costs $50 for each puppy   (b) it costs $50 for a piece of a puppy

3. (a) the guest wants hotel quarters that have a bedroom and bathroom   (b) give the guest a room and then bathe him

4. (a) you look familiar   (b) her face has been located in places other than between her ears

5. (a) did you join your son at the airport   (b) did you encounter your son for the first time ever at the airport

6. (a) Charles can sing "The Star-Spangled Banner" over and over again for a very long time   (b) Richard can sing the song entitled "Stars and Stripes Forever"

7. (a) if you pay a quarter, how much birdseed can you buy   (b) what's the quantity of birdseed needed to feed a quarter.

8. (a) where in England   (b) what part of Annie's body was born in England

9. (a) if you commit the crime, you will be sentenced to live in Alabama for 20 years; if you commit the crime in Alabama, you'll be sentenced to 20 years in prison   (b) the words *in Alabama* can be interpreted in two ways

10. (a) so many people are hit by cars that if you averaged it out, it would come to one person every five minutes   (b) the same person is being hit repeatedly by a car every five minutes

Switching Sounds or Words

11. (a) *trains to run* and *runs to trains*   (b) *trains to run*—learns how to move quickly; *runs to trains*—moves quickly to catch trains   (c) because marathon runners have to run as part of their training and commuters often have to run quickly to catch a train

12. (a) *runs for home* and *home run*   (b) *runs for home*—moving quickly to get home; *home run*—baseball hit out of the ballpark   (c) being late for dinner would cause a boy to run, and when a ball is hit out of the ballpark, it is considered a home run

13. (a) *cast of hundreds* and *hundreds of casts*   (b) *cast of hundreds*—200 or more people appearing in a movie; *hundreds of casts*—200 or more plaster bandages that are used to set broken bones   (c) motion pictures have a set of players called a *cast;* people at a ski resort sometimes, while skiing, break a bone, which requires a cast in order to heal properly

14. (a) *go to the seas* and *cease to go*   (b) *go to the seas*—sail away in a ship; *cease to go*—stop working

15. (a) *weak one* and *one week*   (b) *weak one*—a person who can hardly stand up; *one week*—seven days   (c) when you are weak, you many have difficulty standing, and seven days compose one week

16. (a) *killed with the cold* and *cold with the kilt*   (b) *killed with the cold*—caused to die from cold weather; *cold with the kilt*—feels the cold temperature because of the skimpy skirt (i.e., kilt) Scotsmen wear

17. (a) *peals/steeple* and *steals/people*   (b) *p* and *st*   (c) a steeple bell peals (i.e., rings) and a pickpocket steals (especially in a crowed place)

18. (a) *living* and *world*   (b) the world owes him a living   (c) the feeling someone has that he or she is entitled to financial security without earning it   (d) to define *environmentalist* (a person who believes people should keep the world healthy and safe)

19. (a) *howls/prairie* and *prowls/hairy*   (b) *h* and *pr*   (c) a coyote lives on a prairie and howls; a flea prowls in the hair of animals

20. (a) *roots for the Yanks* and *yanks for the roots*   (b) *roots for the Yanks*—to cheer for the New York Yankees baseball team; *yanks for the roots*—to remove a tooth, making sure to get the roots too   (c) people root for baseball teams, like the Yankees, and dentists have to pull hard (yank) to remove teeth

RED

Stress and Pausing Changes

21. (a) *bar tender*   (b) bartender   (c) a person who mixes and serves drinks   (d) bar tinder—the wood that constructs the bar

22. (a) *ex-stream*   (b) extreme—of the highest degree   (c) it no longer has water in it

23. (a) mini mum   (b) a tiny, dead creature preserved in wraps   (c) *very small mummy*

24. (a) holly would   (b) the leaves and berries of an evergreen tree would grow there   (c) *Christmas trees*

25. (a) an exclamation of surprise or displeasure   (b) dog gone   (c) *puppy ran away*

26. (a) an apple is   (b) *fruit*

27. (a) you go first   (b) *Over the Cliff*

28. (a) no bell   (b) *disconnect his doorbell*

29. (a) *want who*   (b) one two   (c) *counting to three*

30. (a) *justice* means fair and laws often attempt to enforce fairness   (b) an ice cube is just a piece of ice

Orange Deck

Sound Changes

1. (a) *jab*   (b) job   (c) *acupuncture*   (d) acupuncture is the Chinese practice of puncturing (i.e., jabbing) the body with needles to effect health benefits; *a jab well done* resembles the expression *a job well done*

2. (a) *Mice*   (b) Rice   (c) *snap, crackle, squeak, Krispies*   (d) "Snap, Crackle, Pop" is part of a jingle in an advertisement for Rice Krispies cereal; mice squeak and *mice* rhymes with *rice*

3. (a) *Grape*   (b) Great   (c) *purple, thousands of miles long, Wall of China*   (d) some grapes are purple and *grape* starts with the same sounds as *great*

4. (a) *whittle*   (b) little   (c) *carve wood*   (d) taking a little off at a time is the best way to carve (whittle) wood; *whittle* rhymes with *little*

5. (a) *mousecarade*   (b) masquerade   (c) *type of party, mice*   (d) *mousecarade*, a type of party for mice, starts and ends with the same syllables as *masquerade*, a type of party for people

6. (a) *chat*   (b) cat   (c) *gossip, out of the bag*   (d) *chat* rhymes with *cat; let the cat out of the bag* means "to tell something that is supposed to be secret," and gossip is talk about other people's secrets

7. (a) *ghost*   (b) coast   (c) *why can't I see it, clear*   (d) it's possible to see through a clear object, *the coast is clear* (i.e., no enemy or danger is in sight) is a familiar expression, and *ghost* rhymes with *coast*

8. (a) *thug*   (b) tug   (c) *big ships fear, push them around*   (d) thugs push people around and *thug* rhymes with *tug*, which is a kind of boat that pulls big ships

9. (a) *pronto-saurus*   (b) brontosaurus   (c) *fast dinosaur*   (d) *pronto* means "fast," and *pronto-saurus* rhymes with *brontosaurus*, which is a dinosaur

10. (a) *Salmon*   (b) Simon   (c) *game, little fish play*   (d) *salmon* is a kind of fish, *salmon* starts and ends with the same sounds as *Simon*, and Simon Says is a game children play

11. (a) *lunge*   (b) lunch   (c) *fencing master, noon*   (d) fencers make quick forward jabs (i.e., lunges) with a sword, and *lunge* starts with the same sounds as *lunch*, which is frequently eaten at noon

12. (a) *Mousekeeping*   (b) Housekeeping   (c) *magazine, cats read*   (d) *Good Mousekeeping* sounds like *Good Housekeeping*, a well-known magazine, and cats are interested in mice

13. (a) *quacker*   (b) cracker   (c) *smart duck*   (d) *wise* can mean *smart*, ducks quack, and *wise quacker* sounds like *wisecracker* (i.e., someone who makes a witty or sarcastic remark)

14. (a) *glowing*   (b) growing   (c) *baby candle, pains*   (d) candles glow, children sometimes get growing pains, and *glow* rhymes with *grow*

15. (a) *diapurrs*   (b) diapers   (c) *baby cats wear*   (d) cats purr and babies wear diapers; *diapurrs* sounds like *diapers*

16. (a) *Kong*   (b) King   (c) *musical comedy, gorilla*   (d) *King Kong* is a movie about a gorilla, *The King and I* is a well-known musical show and film, and *Kong* starts and ends with the same sounds as *King*

17. (a) *boa*   (b) boy   (c) *snake, bouncing baby*   (d) a boa is a kind of snake, people often refer to a newborn male as *a bouncing baby boy*, and *boa* starts with the same sounds as *boy*

18. (a) *stocky*   (b) stock   (c) *health-food store, Wall Street, brokers*   (d) *stocky* is another word for *overweight*, Wall Street brokers deal with stocks, and *stocky* starts with the same syllable as *stock*

ORANGE

19. (a) *Ro-meow*   (b) Romeo   (c) *cat's, play, Juliet*   (d) cats meow, Romeo and Juliet is a well-known play, and *Ro-meow* starts with the same sounds as *Romeo*

20. (a) *Hounda*   (b) Honda   (c) *dog's, car*   (d) a dog is sometimes called a *hound*, and *Hounda* starts and ends with the same sounds as *Honda* (i.e., a kind of car)

21. (a) *purr*   (b) poor   (c) *cats, rich*   (d) the opposite of *rich* is *poor*, and *poor* starts and ends with the same sounds as *purr*, which is what cats do

22. (a) *show-arf*   (b) show off   (c) *prize-winning dog*   (d) a dog who is a prizewinner in a show and says "arf" is being called a *show-arf*, which starts and ends with the same sounds as *show off* (i.e., to display nicely for people to see)

23. (a) *hippopotamouse*   (b) hippopotamus   (c) *tiny hippo*   (d) a mouse is tiny compared to a hippo (i.e., hippopotamus), so a small hippo is being called a *hippopotamouse*

24. (a) *thore, thaddle, thilly*   (b) sore, saddle, silly   (c) *Thunder God, horse*   (d) *Thor*, which rhymes with *sore*, is the name of the Thunder God in Norse mythology; a person can become sore when riding a horse without a saddle; the horse mispronounced all of the *s*'s, changing them to *th*'s

25. (a) *copcake*   (b) cupcake   (c) *bake, police officer, birthday*   (d) a police officer is sometimes called a *cop*, and *copcake* sounds like *cupcake*, which can be baked for someone's birthday

26. (a) *mice*   (b) nice   (c) *friendly cats*   (d) cats like to catch mice, and *have a mice day* (i.e., catch some mice today) resembles the saying *have a nice day*, which is what friendly people often say to each other

27. (a) *plot*   (b) pot   (c) *best-selling novel*   (d) a novel has a *plot*, which sounds like *pot*, and a best-seller would make lots of money, which could be called *a pot of gold*

28. (a) *Meringue-utans*   (b) orangutans   (c) *apes, lemon pie*   (d) an orangutan is an ape and meringue is often put on top of a lemon pie; *meringue-utans* rhymes with *orangutans*

29. (a) *Maybe*   (b) Moby   (c) *large white whale, Dick*   (d) *maybe*, which means a person's mind is not made up yet, sounds like *Moby*, and *Moby Dick* is a well-known story about a white whale

30. (a) *crookies*   (b) cookies   (c) *outlaws, dessert*   (d) an outlaw is a crook, and *crookies* rhymes with *cookies*, which are often eaten for dessert

Blue Deck

Challenge Activities

Many responses to these items will vary. The facilitator must judge the appropriateness of all responses. The answer key is merely meant to suggest some possibilities.

1. (a) *brimming pools*   (b) her eyes were filled with tears that were about to roll down her cheeks

2. (a) *proud as a peacock*   (b) Maggie had high self-esteem; she was feeling accomplished (the way a peacock seems as it struts around with its tail feathers fanned)

3. (a) *an open book*   (b) Tara is easy to understand

4. (a) *eats like a bird*   (b) Beth eats very little   (c) Beth eats a lot (like a vulture)

5. Psst! Can you keep a secret?"

6. Drawings will vary.

7. (a) *a face in the crowd*   (b) suggesting someone blends in with the others in a group without making a noticeable impression; there is a face icon in place of the letter *o* in the word *crowd*

8. (a) *a cat has nine lives*   (b) *octo* is another way of saying *eight,* and *puss* is another word for *cat*

9. (a) *blocks of ice*   (b) Arthur's feet were very cold

10. (a) *burned his bridges*   (b) he made decisions that can't be changed in the future; he left himself no way to escape   (c) *bridges* is changed to *britches*   (d) *britches* is another word for *pants,* and the camper's pants were burned when he backed into a campfire; *britches* rhymes with *bridges*

11. (a) *if you play with fire, you may get burned*   (b) if you take a big risk or try something dangerous, you may get into trouble

12. (a) she just sat there without acting or responding   (b) he or she might be sick, tired, or not have the knowledge or interest to act, move, or respond

13. Drawings will vary.

14. (a) pain in the neck   (b) an obnoxious or annoying person or event; the letters that spell the word *pain* are placed within the letters that spell the word *neck*

15. (a) the cat's fur was shiny and soft   (b) the cow's tail was like a whip; the fish seemed to move like a dart

16. (a) double parked   (b) when two cars are parked side-by-side with one of them blocking a lane of traffic; the word *parked* is written twice in a row (i.e., double)

17. (a) you're in my way   (b) you are preventing me from reaching my goal or from getting to where I'm going; the word *you're* is written in between the words *my* and *way*

18. (a) *popsicle stick*   (b) Jake was tall and thin.

19. (a) bulb   (b) *florist, light up, garden, plant*

20. (a) too big for its britches   (b) too haughty for one's status or age; disdainfully proud

21. (a) *look like a million bucks*   (b) you look wonderful; you look like a large pile of money

22. (a) Are you sure? and Where am I now?   (b) *Hopelessly Lost*

23. Drawings will vary.

24. (a) Theo looked bedraggled and worn   (b) Carmine looked like the cat that swallowed the canary; Jamie looked like she'd just seen a ghost

25. (a) *on the other hand*   (b) one hand would be warm, and the other hand would be cold   (c) an alternate way of looking at things; an alternate possibility

26. (a) *foot*   (b) a measurement of 12 inches; the end part of a leg upon which people stand   (c) a yard (i.e., three feet in length)

27. "Knock-knock." "Who's there?" "Betty." "Betty who?" "Betty will slip if he steps on the banana peel."

28. (a) call before you come   (b) call ahead to let the person know you are coming; the word *call* is written ahead of the words *you* and *come*

29. (a) did you let   (b) *the cat out*

30. (a) *Are you a man or a mouse?*   (b) are you a person or a rodent   (c) are you brave or a coward

References

Abrahamsen, E.P., and Sprouse, P.T. (1995). Fable comprehension by children with learning disabilities. *Journal of Learning Disabilities, 28,* 302–308.

Arnold, K., and Hornett, D. (1990). Teaching idioms to children who are deaf. *Teaching Exceptional Children, 22,* 14–17.

Ball, E.W. (1997). Phonological awareness: Implications for whole language and emergent literacy programs. *Topics in Language Disorders, 17*(3), 14–26.

Brown, G., Anderson, A., Shillcock, R., and Yule, G. (1984). *Teaching talk.* New York: Cambridge University Press.

Catts, H.W. (1999). Phonological awareness: Putting research into practice. *Special Interest Division 1: Language Learning and Education.* Rockville, MD: ASHA.

Clarke-Klein, S.M. (1994). Expressive phonological deficiencies: Impact on spelling development. *Topics in Language Disorders, 14*(2), 40–55.

Donahue, M., and Bryan, T. (1984). Communicative skills and peer relations of learning disabled adolescents. *Topics in Language Disorders, 4*(2), 10–21.

Gillon, G., and Dodd, B. (1995). The effects of training phonological, semantic, and syntactic processing skills in spoken language on reading ability. *Language, Speech, and Hearing Services in Schools, 26,* 58–68.

Green, T.A., and Pepicello, W.J. (1978). Wit in riddling: A linguistic perspective. *Genre, 11,* 1–13.

Honeck, R.P., Voegtle, K., Dorfmueller, M.A., and Hoffman, R.R. (1980). Proverbs, meaning, and group structure. In R.P. Honeck and R.R. Hoffman (Eds.), *Cognition and figurative language* (pp. 127–161). Hillsdale, NJ: Erlbaum.

Larson, V. L., and McKinley, N. (1995). *Language disorders in older students: Preadolescents and adolescents.* Eau Claire, WI: Thinking Publications.

Lloyd, P. (1994). Referential communication: Assessment and intervention. *Topics in Language Disorders, 14*(3), 55–69.

MacDonald, G.W., and Cornwall, A. (1995). The relationship between phonological awareness and reading and spelling achievement eleven years later. *Journal of Learning Disabilities, 28,* 523–527.

Milosky, L.M. (1990). The role of world knowledge in language comprehension and language intervention. *Topics in Language Disorders, 10*(3), 1–13.

Nelson, N.W. (1993). *Childhood language disorders in context: Infancy through adolescence.* New York: Macmillan.

Nicolosi, L., Harryman, E., and Kresheck, J. (1996). *Terminology of communication disorders* (4th ed.). Baltimore: Williams and Wilkins.

Nippold, M.A. (1985). Comprehension of figurative language in youth. *Topics in Language Disorders, 5*(3), 1–20.

Nippold, M.A. (1991). Evaluating and enhancing idiom comprehension in language disordered students. *Language, Speech, and Hearing Services in Schools, 22,* 100–106.

Nippold, M.A. (1998). *Later language development: The school-age and adolescent years* (2nd ed.). Austin, TX: ProEd.

Nippold, M.A., Allen, M.M., and Kirsch, D.I. (2000). How adolescents comprehend unfamiliar proverbs: The role of top-down and bottom-up processes. *Journal of Speech and Hearing Research, 43,* 621–630.

Nippold, M.A., Allen, M.M., and Kirsch, D.I. (2001). Proverb comprehension as a function of reading proficiency in preadolescents. *Language, Speech, and Hearing Services in Schools, 32,* 90–100.

Nippold, M.A., and Fey, S.H. (1983). Metaphoric understanding in preadolescents having a history of language acquisition difficulties. *Language, Speech, and Hearing Services in Schools, 14,* 171–180.

Nippold, M.A., Hegel, S.L., Sohlberg, M.M., and Schwarz, I.E. (1999). Defining abstract entities: Development in pre-adolescents, adolescents, and young adults. *Journal of Speech, Language, and Hearing Research, 42,* 473–481.

Nippold, M.A., and Martin, S.T. (1989). Idiom interpretation in isolation versus context: A developmental study with adolescents. *Journal of Speech and Hearing Research, 32,* 59–66.

Nippold, M.A., Martin, S.T., and Erskine, B. (1988). Proverb comprehension in context: A developmental study with children and adolescents. *Journal of Speech and Hearing Research, 31,* 19–28.

Nippold, M.A., and Rudzinski, M. (1993) Familiarity and transparency in idiom explanations: A developmental study of children and adolescents. *Journal of Speech and Hearing Research, 36,* 728–737.

Pepicello, W.J. (1980). Linguistic strategies in riddling. *Western Folklore, 39,* 1–16.

Piaget, J. (1954). *The construction of reality in the child.* New York: Basic Books.

Secord, W.A., and Wiig, E.H. (1993). Interpreting figurative language expressions. *Folia Phoniatrica, 45*, 1–9.

Seidenberg, P.L. (1988). Cognitive and academic instructional intervention for learning-disabled adolescents. *Topics in Language Disorders, 8*(3), 56–71.

Snow, C., Cancini, H., Gonzalez, P., and Shriberg E. (1989). Giving formal definitions: An oral language correlate of school literacy. In D. Bloome (Ed.), *Classrooms and literacy* (pp. 233–249). Norwood, NJ: Ablex.

Spector, C.C. (1990). Linguistic humor comprehension of normal and language-impaired adolescents. *Journal of Speech and Hearing Disorders, 55*, 533–541.

Spector, C.C. (1992). Remediating humor comprehension deficits in language-impaired students. *Language, Speech and Hearing Services in Schools, 23*, 20–27.

Spector, C.C. (1996). Children's comprehension of idioms in the context of humor. *Language, Speech, and Hearing Services in Schools, 27*, 307–313.

Spector, C.C. (1997). *Saying one thing, meaning another: Activities for clarifying ambiguous language.* Eau Claire, WI: Thinking Publications.

Spector, C.C. (1999). *Sound effects: Activities for developing phonological awareness.* Eau Claire, WI: Thinking Publications.

van Kleeck, A. (1984). Metalinguistic skills: Cutting across spoken and written language and problem-solving abilities. In G. Wallach and K. Butler (Eds.), *Language learning disabilities in school-age children* (pp. 128–153). Baltimore: Williams and Wilkins.

Vygotsky, L.S. (1962). *Thought and language.* Cambridge, MA: MIT Press.

Watson, R. (1985). Towards a theory of definition. *Journal of Child Language, 12*, 181–197.

Wiig, E.H., and Semel, E.M. (1984). Language assessment and intervention for the learning disabled. Columbus, OH: Merrill.

Wiig, E.H., and Wiig, K.M. (1999). *On conceptual learning.* Retrieved August 22, 2001 from http://www.krii.com/articles.htm